Women's Health Case Studies

Rebecca K. Donohue, PhD, RN, CS
Assistant Professor, Simmons College
Graduate School for Health Studies, Graduate Nursing
Nurse Practitioner, Simmons College Student Health Service
Boston, Massachusetts

Deborah A. Morrill, MPH, RN, CS
Nurse Practitioner, Marino Center for Progressive Health
Cambridge, Massachusetts

Carol Tallon, MS, RN, CS
Nurse Practitioner, Fresh Pond Women's Health
Cambridge, Massachusetts

APPLETON & LANGE
Stamford, Connecticut

Notice: The authors and the publisher of this volume have taken care to make certain that the doses of drugs and schedules of treatment are correct and compatible with the standards generally accepted at the time of publication. Nevertheless, as new information becomes available, changes in treatment and in the use of drugs become necessary. The reader is advised to carefully consult the instruction and information material included in the package insert of each drug or therapeutic agent before administration. This advice is especially important when using, administering, or recommending new or infrequently used drugs. The authors and publisher disclaim all responsibility for any liability, loss, injury, or damage incurred as a consequence, directly or indirectly, of the use and application of any of the contents of this volume.

www.appletonlange.com

99 00 01 02 / 11 10 9 8 7 6 5 4 3 2 1

Prentice Hall International (UK) Limited, *London*
Prentice Hall of Australia Pty. Limited, *Sydney*
Prentice Hall Canada, Inc., *Toronto*
Prentice Hall Hispanoamericana, S.A., *Mexico*
Prentice Hall of India Private Limited, *New Delhi*
Prentice Hall of Japan, Inc., *Tokyo*
Simon & Schuster Asia Pte. Ltd., *Singapore*
Editora Prentice Hall do Brasil Ltda., *Rio de Janeiro*
Prentice Hall, *Upper Saddle River, New Jersey*

Library of Congress Cataloging-in-Publication Data
Donohue, Rebecca K.
    Women's health case studies / Rebecca K. Donohue, Deborah A.
Morrill, Carol Tallon.
        p.   cm. — (Nurse practitioner certification review series)
    Includes bibliographical references and index.
    ISBN 0-8385-9819-6 (pbk. : alk. paper)
    1. Nurse practitioners—Examinations, questions, etc.   2. Women—
Diseases—Examinations, questions, etc.   3. Women—Health and
hygiene—Examinations, questions, etc.   4. Gynecologic nursing—
Examinations, questions, etc.   5. Maternity nursing—Examinations,
questions, etc.   I. Morrill, Deborah A.   II. Tallon, Carol.
III. Title.   IV. Series.
    [DNLM: 1. Genital Diseases, Female—nursing examination questions.
2. Nurse Practitioners examination questions.   3. Obstetrical
Nursing examination questions.   4. Women's Health examination
questions.   WY 18.2 D687w 1999]
RT82.8.D66   1999
610.73'678'076—dc21
DNLM/DLC
for Library of Congress   98-17718
                                        CIP

Editor-in-Chief: Sally J. Barhydt
Production Editor: Karen Davis
Cover Designer: Libby Schmitz

ISBN 0-8385-9819-6

PRINTED IN THE UNITED STATES OF AMERICA

Contents

To our husbands—

Chuck Koeniger
Robert Carroll
Paul Tallon

To our collective children—

Brendan, Paul, & Nicholas Koeniger
Tyler & Alexandra Carroll
Laura & Paul Tallon

Our grateful thanks for patience and understanding during the hours of labor spent writing this book. Although this meant missing a few bedtime stories, hockey games, and family outings, it allowed our children to see work in progress and the evolution of a goal shared by three mothers with a vision.

Preface

This book is designed to help you prepare for the Women's Health Nurse Practitioner Certification exam. To do this, we have provided real-life case studies and over 400 questions covering the content likely to be tested in the actual exam. The case studies in this book are divided into four content areas that you will encounter in the National Certification Corporation (NCC) exam: gynecology, obstetrics, primary care, and professional issues. The book may therefore be used to determine overall competence in women's health as well as to identify a specific content area needing additional concentration. References included at the back of the book provide a further study resource.

The answers and, perhaps more importantly, the rationales for the correct or best answers are also included. Some answers provide necessary general information, such as a review of breast cancer risk factors or causes of chronic pelvic pain. These items are listed in the table of contents in the Gynecology Answers and Rationales.

Since no book can quite give you the feel of a computerized exam, our objective is to help you review material and information you often see in practice or should be aware of for the exam. You will find that the majority of the questions are linked to "real" cases and concerns across the life span. This offers you an opportunity to delve into a subject and consider what you would do, given the parameters of a particular patient's life at a particular moment in time. Although an attempt was made to fit the material into the content areas of the Women's Health exam to allow you to identify your strengths and weaknesses in one area, in real life it may be difficult to distinguish a gynecologic visit from a primary care visit. And of course the certification exam itself will offer questions in random order and subject.

As students, faculty, and nurse practitioners, we have seen the need for a certification review book using the case study approach. We hope that after studying these cases and questions you will feel confident of your preparation, ready to take the certification exam and to begin your practice. We welcome your comments and your feedback, which can only improve our efforts in the future.

Rebecca K. Donohue
Deborah A. Morrill
Carol Tallon

About the Women's Health Nurse Practitioner Exam

The Women's Health Nurse Practitioner Certification exam is offered by the National Certification Corporation (NCC) of the Obstetric, Gynecologic, and Neonatal Specialties. The exam itself consists of a minimum of 150 questions in computerized format. Some questions have illustrations or figures, and sometimes a number of questions are based on one case situation.

The exam content is divided unequally among gynecology (40–45%), obstetrics (35–40%), primary care (20–25%), and professional issues (less than 5%). We have tried to reflect that in the more than 400 questions in this book. Unlike the exam, the questions here are grouped by the major subject areas, recognizing that some areas of medicine and nursing cross these arbitrary boundaries and could have been placed in different sections. We have also relied more heavily on cases than you may find in the actual exam. We felt this would help you study more thoroughly and realistically, especially if certain elements have not been as well represented in your particular practice or educational program.

You are required to answer all the questions, but you may mark questions and return to those needing further pondering within the time allowed. A minimum of 10 unidentified questions will be pretested for possible inclusion in future exams; they will not count toward your final score.

GENERAL EXAM INFORMATION

To obtain an application, contact NCC at:

645 North Michigan Avenue, Suite 900
Chicago, IL 60611
or call (312) 951-0207

On receipt of your applications, NCC will send you a *Guide* to the examination that contains a content outline for the exam, a suggested bibliography, and additional information about the exam process. NCC will notify you of your eligibility status within 4 weeks after receiving your application.

You must take the exam within 90 days after being granted admission to the exam or forfeit your fees. The exam will be given to you at the nearest Sylvan Technology Center. Contact Sylvan to set up your appointment to take the test.

Your exam is scored and analyzed within 10 days after your exam date. You will receive your score report and be notified of your pass or fail status. Successful candidates also receive further information about how to maintain their certification.

HELPFUL HINTS

This exam is not like the NCLEX computer-adaptive test: you must answer all the questions on the exam since the exam will not stop once you have hit the "pass" mark. But your exam is computer sorted, so your exam will be different from that of others taking the same test on the same day and may reflect different content area percentages.

Choose the best response. There is only one correct answer for each question. If you do not know an answer, give your best guess. There is no penalty for guessing because your score is based on the total number of questions you answer correctly.

Don't cram the night before. Get a good night's rest, have a big glass of orange juice one hour before the exam, and go easy on the caffeine.

We wish you GOOD LUCK!

Rebecca, Deb, and Carol

I

Gynecology

Gynecology Cases and Questions

Questions 1–4

Lisa is a 27-year-old graduate student who presents at your office for an annual visit. She denies any medication or drug use, has no acute symptoms, and is in a monogamous relationship of 5 years' duration. She admits to significant stress that seems to become unmanageable the week or 10 days prior to her menstrual period. She complains of irritability, emotional tension, breast tenderness, and food cravings. She also notes inability to concentrate and forgetfulness. Her LNMP was 2 weeks ago and her cycles are every 28 days with cramping on the first day of menstrual bleeding. Her family and personal history is negative for depression and mood disorders. She admits to resolution of all symptoms upon onset of menses.

1. What are important indicators in diagnosing Premenstrual Syndrome?

   (A) Symptoms of mood changes, changes in appetite, food cravings, breast tenderness, weight gain, and arthralgias
   (B) The symptoms are present in the follicular and luteal phase often resolving within 1–2 days of bleeding
   (C) The symptoms are not apparent in women who have had a hysterectomy

2. What is the "gold standard" for validation of Premenstrual Syndrome?

   (A) Complete detailed history of symptoms, physical exam, and Pap smear
   (B) Laboratory tests to rule out other medical disorders
   (C) Patient keeps a daily symptom diary for 2–3 months

3. What recommendations might be initially suggested for this patient?

   (A) Advise regular exercise for at least 30 minutes per day and increase intake of fresh foods and avoid refined and highly processed foods. Decrease salt, sugar, caffeine and fat intake.
   (B) Prescribe Prozac 10 mg po daily.
   (C) Prescribe progesterone 100 mg po in AM and 200 mg po hs 10–14 days before menses.

4. What recommendations are most appropriate as a first step in management of mastalgia?

   (A) Spironolactone therapy
   (B) Danocrine therapy
   (C) Dietary changes to decrease salt, refined sugar, and caffeine intake and to add vitamin E supplements

Questions 5–9

Jennie, 17 years old, wants to start oral contraceptives (OCs). Her past medical history is significant for acne, dysmenorrhea, and mild obesity. Her family history is positive for a mother with adult onset diabetes mellitus (AODM) and father with an myocardial infarction (MI) at age 53. She does not smoke. Menses are regular q 28 days.

5. What is the best oral contraceptive choice for this client?

   (A) Ovral
   (B) Loestrin 1/20 Fe
   (C) Oral contraceptives are contraindicated

6. Recommended screening lab tests before starting client on OCs include

   (A) Fasting cholesterol screen and blood sugar
   (B) Liver function tests
   (C) Thyroid screen

7. While instructing the patient about starting OCs you advise her to take the first pill

   (A) On day one of her menses
   (B) The first Sunday after her menses begins
   (C) Anytime during her cycle

8. You start the patient on a low-dose OC. She experiences break-through bleeding during her first pill cycle. How would you manage the client?

   (A) Provide support and reassurance.
   (B) Change her to another OC.
   (C) Discontinue the OC.

9. In counseling the client about expected changes in her menstrual cycle while on OCs, you would advise her menses will be

   (A) Lighter in flow
   (B) Without change in flow
   (C) Heavier in flow

Questions 10–14

Mrs. Gordon phones your office to make an appointment for her 14-year-old daughter who had her first menses 6 months ago and no cyclical bleeding since that time until 2 days ago. She is presently bleeding heavily, using one to two pads per hour, and feeling lightheaded and dizzy. She has no history of medication or vitamin use, is not sexually active, and has no history of chronic disease or a bleeding disorder.

10. What is the probable cause of dysfunctional uterine bleeding (DUB) in this patient?

    (A) Immaturity or failure of the pituitary gland and hypothalamus with no elevation of the gonadotrophins
    (B) Ovarian failure with a rise in FSH and LH levels

    (C) Unopposed progesterone and the subsequent response of endometrial bleeding

11. Anovulatory bleeding can be attributed to which of the following?

    (A) Chronic illness
    (B) Vitamin deficiency
    (C) Depression

12. What are the symptoms of dysfunctional uterine bleeding?

    (A) Monthly intervals of menstrual bleeding lasting greater than 10 days in duration
    (B) Complete irregular unpredictable bleeding
    (C) Premenstrual molimina and dysmenorrhea

13. Polycystic ovarian disease (PCOD) is also associated with dysfunctional uterine bleeding. This syndrome is characterized by which of the following?

    (A) Hyperandrogenism
    (B) Diabetes mellitus
    (C) Infrequent ovulatory cycles

14. The initial assessment of this adolescent patient with possible dysfunctional uterine bleeding should include determination of blood loss. What should be considered as part of the routine assessment?

    (A) Speculum and bimanual examination
    (B) Endometrial biopsy
    (C) Pelvic ultrasound

Questions 15–19

Helen is a 25-year-old gravida 0 para 0 woman who presents to discuss contraceptive options. Her gynecologic history includes menarche at age 15, menstrual intervals of 26 days, with 5 days of moderate bleeding and dysmenorrhea on days 1 and 2 relieved by Advil. She is not in a monogamous relationship and last intercourse was 2 months ago. A Pap smear result of low-grade squamous intraepithelial neoplasia in 1995 was evaluated by colposcopy and results were normal. She has not had a Pap since that time. Prior contraceptive methods include pills, condoms, and the sponge. She has heard about Depo-Provera and asks your opinion about it.

15. What is the mechanism of action of Depo-Provera?

   (A) Suppression of LH and FSH at the level of the hypothalamus and pituitary and alteration of the endometrium and cervical mucus, producing barriers to implantation and sperm penetration
   (B) Releases consistent levels of levonorgestrel, leading to contraceptive efficacy similiar to sterilization
   (C) Complete suppression of estrogen

16. What are the advantages of Depo-Provera?

   (A) Can be considered for patients with sickle cell anemia and a prior history of thromboembolic event
   (B) Can be used in the treatment of dysfunctional uterine bleeding
   (C) Causes an increase in bone density

17. What is the correct dose for administering this contraceptive?

   (A) Depo-Provera 150 mg/mL deep gluteal or deltoid every 3 months
   (B) Depo-Provera 100 mg/mL SQ every 3 months
   (C) Calculate the dose according to the patient's body weight to maximize contraceptive impact given at 3-month intervals

18. Helen's history raises some important concerns. What counseling must be included prior to proceeding with the Depo-Provera injection?

   (A) Psychotherapy consult to assess emotional status and risk of depression
   (B) Need to resolve Pap smear status prior to Depo-Provera contraception
   (C) Discussion of the action, side effects, and risks of Depo-Provera prior to using the method and the need to use added protection to decrease sexually transmitted–disease risk

19. Helen returns for her second injection 16 weeks following the initial dose. What is the appropriate management in this case?

   (A) Identify last menstrual period and perform urine HCG and pelvic exam. If negative, give Depo-Provera injection.
   (B) Await onset of menses and advise condoms and foam until then.
   (C) Document bleeding dates and draw serum HCG. Give Depo-Provera if HCG is negative.

Questions 20–23

A multiparous monogamous client requests a diaphragm fitting.

20. What would represent a contraindication to this method for her?

   (A) Pelvic relaxation
   (B) Irregular menses
   (C) Chronic urinary tract infection (UTI)

21. Which of the following diaphragm types would you select for a client with pelvic relaxation?

   (A) Wide-seal, flat-spring rim
   (B) Coil-spring rim
   (C) Arching-spring rim

22. In addition to providing informed consent and insertion instruction to this client for diaphragm use, you provide information on

   (A) STD risk
   (B) Postcoital emergency contraception
   (C) Tubal sterilization

23. A postpartum breastfeeding client wants to use LAM (lactation amenorrhea method) as a temporary method of contraception. What advice would you give her?

   (A) Begin using another method of contraception once menses resumes.
   (B) Bottle feeding may be used to supplement while weaning.
   (C) LAM is not effective.

Questions 24–25

A single 37-year-old female gravida 2 para 0 therapeutic AB ×2 not currently in a bilaterally monogamous relationship requests an IUD insertion. She has mild dysmenorrhea with heavy periods (menorrhagia). She says she does not want children, nor does she want a tubal sterilization. The client has no insurance and is not currently in a relationship.

24. You would first tell the client about

(A) Cu T 380A IUD (Paragard)
(B) Progesterone T (Progestasert system)
(C) The full informed consent

25. The client has a Cu T 380A IUD inserted. The most common reported nuisance side effects of the copper IUD are menstrual cramping and spotting, increased mucus discharge, and

(A) Ectopic pregnancy
(B) PID
(C) Increased menstrual flow

Questions 26–28

A young woman seeks information and advice on the polyurethane Reality® female condom. You also discuss the various barrier contraceptive methods with her.

26. About the Reality® condom, you tell her

(A) It can be inserted immediately before intercourse or up to 8 hours before intercourse
(B) It should be used with a male condom for greater efficacy
(C) She may not use oil-based lubricants as the polyurethane will deteriorate

27. Which method would require the least amount of planning ahead?

(A) Female condom
(B) Diaphragm
(C) Cervical cap

28. The female condom as a female-controlled barrier method is an important option for this client as it

(A) Provides contraceptive protection
(B) Provides STD protection
(C) Both A and B

Questions 29–33

29. A patient asks about the various over-the-counter contraceptives available. The following statements are true regarding contraceptive foam, jelly, tablets and cream EXCEPT

(A) Vaginal contraceptive foam protection is immediate and remains effective for at least 1 hour.
(B) Contraceptive protection of contraceptive jellies and creams is immediate and remains effective for at least 1 hour.
(C) Protection of contraceptive suppositories and tablets is immediate and remains effective for at least 1 hour.

30. Spermicides _____ STD risk and have been associated with a(n) _____ in cervical cancer

(A) Decrease, increase
(B) Decrease, decrease
(C) Increase, decrease

31. The active ingredient in spermicides is

(A) Propylene glycol
(B) Nonoxynol-9
(C) Imidazole

32. Comparing the efficacy of spermicides for typical use versus near-perfect use, the percentage of women experiencing an accidental pregnancy within the first year of use would be

(A) Typical use, 21%; perfect use, 6%
(B) Typical use, 12%; perfect use, 3%
(C) Typical use, 36%; perfect use, 20%

33. Common errors of patients who use contraceptive foam are

(A) Failing to use another applicator with each act of intercourse
(B) Using too much foam with each act of intercourse
(C) Shaking the foam can too vigorously

Questions 34–36

34. In providing patient education about male condoms, you advise that

    (A) Latex condoms have been shown to be effective against pregnancy and STDs

    (B) "Skins" are as effective as latex condoms in preventing pregnancy and STDs

    (C) Latex condoms can be used with oil-based lubricants

35. The single most important message to give regarding condom use is

    (A) Do not use condoms with a cervical cap

    (B) Do not use condoms with a diaphragm and vaginal gel

    (C) Use the condoms correctly and consistently

36. If a condom has torn (or slipped off)

    (A) Immediately insert spermicidal foam or gel into the vagina

    (B) Go to the emergency room

    (C) Switch to another method

Questions 37–39

Deena has an appointment to discuss contraceptive options. She is 8 weeks postpartum and breastfeeding. She notices stress incontinence when coughing and exercising.

37. The pelvic examination reveals a first-degree cystocele. Which choice of contraception would *not* be suitable for this patient?

    (A) Cervical cap

    (B) Flat-spring diaphragm

    (C) IUD

38. The patient is fitted for a cervical cap. The clinician reviews the instructions. Which statement is true concerning cervical cap use?

    (A) The patient should fill the cervical cap ⅓ with spermicide and insert one applicatorful prior to each intercourse.

    (B) If the patient notes dislodgment, she should replace the cap on the cervix and phone you within 72 hours for postcoital contraception.

    (C) The initial follow-up visit is scheduled in 3 months to assess cap fit and success and to repeat the Pap smear.

39. The most important step in assessing cervical cap success is the following:

    (A) Assure proper placement by checking for location of the cervix within the cap and assessing degree of suction of the cervical cap rim.

    (B) Insertion of the cap should occur at least 1 hour before intercourse.

    (C) The patient should check for cervical cap dislodgment following intercourse.

Questions 40–46

Natasha, a 36-year-old G0 P0, requests information about Norplant contraception. She has a history of menarche at age 12 years and 27-day intervals between 5-day cycles of menstrual bleeding. She is a smoker, has annual gynecologic exams, and a normal Pap smear history. She has used oral contraceptives in the past and discontinued because of depression. She has a history of infrequent migraines that are relieved by nonsteroidal antiinflammatory drugs and relaxation. She is in a monogamous relationship and desires to postpone having a family for 5 years while in a doctoral program but will be planning a pregnancy immediately following Norplant removal. Her medical history is negative for absolute contraindications associated with hormonal contraception. She understands that irregular bleeding cycles are one of the common side effects of Norplant but does not think it will interfere with her lifestyle.

40. What is the most common reason women discontinue Norplant in the first year of use?

    (A) Weight gain

    (B) Depression

    (C) Unpredictable bleeding

41. Natasha's history of depression warrants further evaluation. After a detailed history is taken what might be an option to assess her response to the use of Norplant?

    (A) Place the patient on 3 cycles of a combined oral contraceptive containing levonorgestrel.
    (B) Place the patient on 3 cycles of Ovrette.
    (C) Place the patient on Depo-Provera for 3 months.

42. Headaches may be associated with Norplant use. What findings indicate an increase in intracranial hypertension?

    (A) Ophthalmoscopic findings of papilledema
    (B) Elevated blood pressure and pulse
    (C) Blurred vision

43. What situation would make Norplant a better option than Depo-Provera for this patient?

    (A) Plans for pregnancy immediately following cessation of contraception
    (B) History of depression
    (C) History of migraine headache

44. What is the most important goal of the Norplant insertion process?

    (A) To avoid causing unnecessary pain to the patient
    (B) To avoid infection at the insertion site
    (C) To ensure proper placement of the implants

45. How would you counsel this patient following Norplant removal in terms of risk of pregnancy?

    (A) Levonorgestrel levels taper off slowly over the next several weeks and pregnancy risk is low.
    (B) Levonorgestrel levels decrease significantly following Norplant removal making pregnancy risk immediate.
    (C) Pregnancy risk is unlikely until the patient has resumed at least 2 normal menstrual cycles.

46. Natasha phones the office complaining of persistent vaginal bleeding of 25 days' duration following Norplant insertion. What treatment would be appropriate for this patient following a complete workup to rule out other causes of bleeding?

    (A) Ibuprofen 600 mg po every 6 hours for 5 days
    (B) Ortho-Novum 1/35 28 days for 3 cycles
    (C) Premarin 2.5 mg po daily for 21 days

Questions 47–51

A young woman comes to the office and explains that she had intercourse the night before and "the condom broke." She asks you what her risk of pregnancy is. She is currently in day 13 of a regular 28-day cycle.

47. You tell her that her risk of becoming pregnant is

    (A) 5–12%
    (B) 60–75%
    (C) 15–26%

48. You discuss postcoital contraception with the client. You would advise her that

    (A) Too much time has elapsed and so treatment will not work
    (B) You will administer Ovral 2 tabs po stat followed by 2 additional tabs 12 hours later
    (C) She must wait a month and see if she gets her period

49. The client asks you how effective the "morning-after" pill is. You tell her it is _____ % effective.

    (A) 25
    (B) >75
    (C) 50

50. During counseling of this client you would advise her that postcoital contraception as a treatment to reduce the risk of pregnancy is most effective when

    (A) The first dose is given as soon as possible
    (B) It is given anytime during the first cycle
    (C) The first dose can be given at 72 hours

51. RU 486 (mifepristone) for early pregnancy termination is not currently available in the United States. RU 486 works by

(A) Blocking the normal action of progesterone
(B) Binding with estrogen
(C) Causing cell lysis

Questions 52–58

A young woman presents with acute onset of dysuria, urgency, and frequency ×1 day. She denies a history of vaginal itching, irritation, or vaginal sores. She has been in a new relationship for 3 months and uses vaginal contraceptive suppositories and condoms for contraception. Her history is significant for increased sexual activity 2 days ago.

52. The acute onset of dysuria is most characteristic of bacteria associated with

(A) Lower urinary tract infection
(B) Vulvitis
(C) Upper urinary tract infection

53. Studies have indicated that spermicide can _____ the risk of bacteriuria.

(A) Increase
(B) Decrease
(C) Have no effect on

54. A sexual history is important in this client with the abrupt onset of dysuria in order to rule out urethritis with

(A) *N. gonorrhoeae*
(B) Chlamydia
(C) Bacterial vaginosis

55. Which urine lab test would you order for this client?

(A) Urine culture and sensitivity
(B) Urinalysis
(C) Follow-up culture in 1 week

56. In confirming the diagnosis of cystitis the urine dipstick would show

(A) Pyuria and bacteriuria
(B) Pyuria
(C) Bacteriuria

57. The organism most commonly associated with acute onset of dysuria is

(A) *Escherichia coli*
(B) *Klebsiella*
(C) *Chlamydia trachomatis*

58. The appropriate antibiotic treatment of this client's cystitis infection would be

(A) Single-dose therapy
(B) 3-day therapy
(C) 7-day regimen

Questions 59–61

Meredith, a 32-year-old G2 P0 AB ×2, comes to your office for an annual examination. Her last exam and Pap smear were 4 years ago. She is a light smoker, has used oral contraceptives for 5 years, and uses a condom with new partners. She is in a monogamous relationship of 1 year's duration. She has no complaints and requests a refill on her birth control pills. She has been studying in Mexico for the past 4 years where oral contraceptives are available without prescription. Her exam is within normal limits. Her cytology returns as atypical squamous cells of undetermined significance (ASCUS). Her gonorrhea, chlamydia, and syphilis screen are negative. When you phone the patient to discuss her results she admits to having had a mild dysplasia on her Pap smear several years before that seemed to resolve without treatment. She does not remember the details of her follow-up plan concerning the prior abnormal Pap smear.

59. What is the next step in the evaluation of her ASCUS Pap smear?

(A) Repeat the Pap smear in 4 months.
(B) Evaluate the patient for evidence of human papilloma virus (HPV) disease by using an acetic-acid wash on the vulva, vagina, and cervix.
(C) Refer the patient for colposcopic evaluation.

60. Which variable in the patient's history would most significantly increase her risk of cervical cancer?

    (A) Smoking
    (B) Oral contraceptive use
    (C) Precursor lesion of the cervix

61. When a patient is exposed to HPV disease by history and clinical evaluation and cytology are normal, what is the next appropriate step in management?

    (A) Order a test to identify viral subtypes that will predict cancer risk.
    (B) Perform an acetic-acid wash and speculoscopy exam.
    (C) Provide counseling on the spectrum of HPV disease, teach the patient genital self-examination and reevaluate in 6 months or sooner if the patient notes symptoms of disease.

Questions 62–67

Paulette, 31 years old G0 P0, consults you about long-term vulvar pain. She has been in a monogamous relationship for 2 years, uses oral contraceptives, has no allergies, and uses no other medications. She appears upset and tearful, verbalizing her lack of hope concerning this chronic pain condition. She describes her pain as burning and rawness, which is exacerbated by touch or pressure. She is unable to use tampons or have intercourse. She cannot wear blue jeans or any constrictive clothing nor ride her bicycle. Review of her medical history elicits a series of candidal vaginitis occurring after a sinus infection 1 year earlier. Treatments included topical terconazole, metronidazole, and steroid creams without resolution of the burning. She denies a history of herpes simplex, genital warts, or sexual abuse. She says she had no pain with sexual activities or touch prior to the symptoms of persistent vulvar burning and rawness.

62. The causes of vulvodynia are unclear and possibly multifactorial. Which entity is not commonly associated with vulvodynia?

    (A) Vulvar vestibulitis
    (B) Vulvar dyesthesia
    (C) Allergic vulvitis

63. What criteria are included when diagnosing vulvar vestibulitis syndrome?

    (A) Chronic or acute pain involving or limited to the vaginal canal
    (B) Severe pain with vestibular touch or pressure including pain with vaginal penetration
    (C) Visible ulcerated lesions identified on colposcopic examination

64. What is the first step in the differential diagnosis of vulvar pain?

    (A) Colposcopic evaluation and biopsies
    (B) Microscopic evaluation of vaginal flora
    (C) Meticulous history taking

65. What chronic pain syndrome may exist with vulvodynia?

    (A) Vulvar intraepithelial neoplasia
    (B) Interstitial cystitis
    (C) Condyloma

66. What is one of the treatment options of vulvodynia?

    (A) 6-month course of Terezol intravaginal cream
    (B) Psychotherapy
    (C) Low-dose tricyclic antidepressant therapy

67. What treatment option would we consider for this client?

    (A) Topical steroids applied topically for 6–12 weeks
    (B) Amitriptyline therapy
    (C) Surgical excision of the vestibular glands

Questions 68–70

Erica returns to your office for an acute care visit. She wants you to evaluate an external rash that she has noticed for the past 2 weeks. She has been in a monogamous relationship for 1 year and has no history of sexually transmitted disease.

68. The clinician examines the patient and notes multiple keratinized growths over the labia

minora and introitus resembling condyloma. What test should be included in her workup?

(A) Vaginal wet mount
(B) Pap smear
(C) Chlamydia culture

69. The patient's menstrual period is 2 weeks late and a urine HCG confirms pregnancy. Which statement is true concerning pregnancy and genital warts?

(A) Treatment with topical therapies will be initiated at 12 weeks' gestation to decrease risk to the fetus.
(B) If the Pap smear is abnormal, colposcopic examination with biopsies and endocervical curettage should be performed.
(C) Laryngeal papillomatosis is a rare but potentially serious consequence of neonatal exposure to the human papilloma virus.

70. What counseling needs to be included to increase the patient's knowledge about this virus?

(A) Condom use with partners will prevent spread of the virus.
(B) Present partners need to be evaluated for lesions but cannot be assumed to be the source of transmission.
(C) Lesion eradication will decrease viral transmission.

Questions 71–76

Alice presents with complaints of persistent vulvar pruritus of 2 months' duration. She is a 56-year-old G3 P3 with her last menstrual period occurring 5 years ago. She is currently taking Premarin 0.625 mg po and Provera 2.5 mg po daily along with 1000 mg po of calcium citrate. She has annual mammograms and physicals and no history of abnormal cytology. She has been in a monogamous relationship for 20 years and has intercourse once a week. She noticed the symptom of genital itching following intercourse. Inspection of the external genitalia reveals thick, symmetrical white lesions occurring bilater-

ally on the labia majora extending posteriorly to the perianal area. The microscopic evaluation of the vaginal secretions is negative for candida, bacteria, and trichomonads.

71. What is true about vulvar dermatoses?

(A) These lesions are often associated with precancerous conditions.
(B) They can be readily managed by surgical excision.
(C) Lichen sclerosus is the most common of these conditions.

72. What characteristics are most commonly associated with lichen sclerosus?

(A) Pruritic, thick gray or white plaques or lesions on the skin or mucosa
(B) Pruritic thin parchment with introital stenosis and atrophic skin changes
(C) Discrete raised hyperpigmented red or brown lesions found on the vulvar and perianal tissue

73. Squamous cell hyperplasia is characterized by a thickened, white, keratinized surface and can be found in isolated areas on the vulva. What is the most common presenting symptom?

(A) Pruritus
(B) Burning
(C) Thickening

74. Mixed dystrophies are present in about 15% of all cases. What is true about this dermatitis?

(A) Mixed dystrophies have a slightly increased rate of atypia as compared to hyperplastic lesions.
(B) Treatment may include steroid treatment to decrease inflammation followed by surgical excision.
(C) This syndrome may be associated with persistent yeast vaginitis.

75. Paget's disease of the vulva may be predictive of underlying adenocarcinomas of the breast and sweat glands and is associated with squamous carcinomas of the vulva and cervix. Other characteristics include the following:

    (A) It is more common in African-American women.
    (B) Often it is clinically misinterpreted as a symptom of vulvar condyloma.
    (C) It presents as a focal velvety, red lesion with sharp, distinct borders.

76. What is the treatment of Paget's disease?

    (A) Trial of testosterone therapy for 6 weeks to see if symptoms and clinical characteristics resolve
    (B) Long-term topical steroid therapy and reevaluations at 3-month intervals
    (C) Surgical excision

Questions 77–83

Linda calls the office in the morning requesting to be seen as soon as possible. She has been up most of the night with abdominal pain, fever, and chills. She has taken Tylenol without significant improvement. When she comes in, she sits bent over and guarding her abdomen, rocking back and forth as she speaks. The clinician begins to question the patient about recent symptoms and events. The patient admits to a new male sexual partner of 2 weeks' duration. She did not use condoms as she felt her birth control pills would protect her from pregnancy and STDs. She admits to increased discharge, dysuria, and postcoital spotting following the last intercourse 5 days ago. Her last menstrual period has just ended. She has felt tired and achy for the past 2–3 days but thought she had the flu. The abdominal pain started yesterday morning and increased in intensity over the last 12 hours.

77. Three clinical symptoms must be present to meet the diagnostic criteria of pelvic inflammatory disease. All the following are essential in meeting these criteria EXCEPT

    (A) Abdominal tenderness
    (B) Cervical motion tenderness
    (C) Purulent cervical discharge

78. The three necessary clinical symptoms have been confirmed by the clinician. Which of the following confirms the diagnosis of PID?

    (A) Elevated sedimentation rate
    (B) Vaginal microscopy finding of excessive white blood cells
    (C) Gram stain of cervical or vaginal discharge showing gram-negative intracellular diplococci

79. Hospitalization is often considered to provide intravenous antibiotic therapy for the patient diagnosed with PID. Which case may be treated using oral antibiotic regimens?

    (A) The patient presents with malaise, temperature of 37°C, and a pelvic mass.
    (B) Patient is HIV positive with a T cell count of 800.
    (C) Patient has cervical motion tenderness, adnexal tenderness, and a thick purulent discharge. Her temperature is 37.5°C.

80. What statement is true concerning gonococcal PID?

    (A) A single episode has no impact on future fertility.
    (B) Transmission is more efficient when the infected carrier is a woman transmitting to the male partner.
    (C) PID symptoms often correlate with a history of a recent menstrual period.

81. PID affects more than one million women annually and is estimated to cost $4.2 billion in yearly expenses. What fact is true concerning this syndrome?

    (A) The infertility sequelae can be avoided with rapid diagnosis and treatment.
    (B) The risk of tubal damage increases with repeated episodes of PID.
    (C) Oral contraceptive and IUD users may have an increased risk of PID.

82. The patient's chlamydia fluorescent antibody test returns positive. What clinical signs are associated with a chlamydial infection?

    (A) Lower abdominal tenderness, fever, and a copious cervical discharge
    (B) Lower abdominal tenderness and a red, friable cervix with or without discharge
    (C) Pelvic pain, fever, arthralgia, and tenosynovitis

83. The clinician performs the examination and palpates the right upper quadrant to assess the liver. She elicits pain and tenderness. Which clinical entity is associated with PID?

   (A) Hepatitis B
   (B) Cholelithiasis
   (C) Fitz-Hugh–Curtis syndrome

Questions 84–88

A 21-year-old college student complains of frothy gray-green vaginal discharge. She is on oral contraceptives and her last coitus was 7 days ago and was associated with diffuse lower abdominal discomfort. LMP was 2 weeks ago. She denies that her male partner has any symptoms.

84. The diagnosis of trichomoniasis can be made on wet prep by

   (A) Motile protozoa with four flagellae and more leukocytes than epithelial cells
   (B) Clue cells with no lactobacilli and no leukocytes
   (C) pH of 5.5 on nitrazine paper

85. Pharmacologic treatment of choice for trichomoniasis is

   (A) Metronidazole (Flagyl)
   (B) Ceftriaxone
   (C) Doxycycline

86. It is not uncommon to have a mixed bacterial vaginal infection. To rule out bacterial vaginosis on wet prep, you would look for

   (A) Clue cells
   (B) Leukocytes
   (C) Bacteria

87. To confirm the diagnosis of bacterial vaginosis (BV), you would look for

   (A) Positive KOH "whiff" test
   (B) Mucopurulent cervicitis
   (C) Positive vaginal culture

88. In the asymptomatic client, pharmacologic treatment _____ be instituted.

   (A) Should
   (B) Should not
   (C) Has not been proven that it should

Questions 89–93

Petra is a 31-year-old G0 P0 with complaints of hot flashes, weight loss, fever, malaise, sore throat pain, and persistent vaginitis. She admits to inconsistent condom use with partners and had a sexual relationship with an IV drug user 3 years ago. She is in a new sexual relationship of 1 month's duration and has not used protection every time. She denies IV drug use, anal intercourse, blood transfusions, and sexual relationships with bisexual men. She admits to a history of herpes genitalis that has increased in frequency this year. A physical exam was performed noting stable vital signs, bilateral axillary lymphadenopathy (>2cm size), and confirmation of candidiasis vaginitis by microscopic exam. Cervicitis was noted and appropriate STD cultures were taken. A Pap smear was taken requesting the cytologist to observe for cellular changes associated with herpes simplex. A 10-lb weight loss was noted from 1 year ago. The patient was counseled on HIV risk and consented to anonymous testing. Her ELISA and Western blot tests returned positive.

89. HIV infects human T lymphocytes of the helper/inducer subset. A CD4 lymphocyte count was ordered for Petra. Her results returned 6000 CD4 cells/mm³ of blood. What drug regimen will be considered for this patient?

   (A) Antiretroviral therapy
   (B) *P. carinii* pneumonia (PCP) prophylaxis
   (C) Prophylactic drug therapy not advised at this time

90. What immunizations should *not* be given at this time?

   (A) Pneumococcal vaccine
   (B) Hepatitis B vaccine
   (C) Polio vaccine

91. Which is a true statement about the risk of gynecologic disease in HIV-positive women?

   (A) HIV-positive women have an increased rate of invasive cervical cancer.
   (B) HIV-positive women have an increased rate of invasive vulvar intraepithelial neoplasia.
   (C) HIV-positive women have an increased rate of cervical intraepithelial neoplasia.

92. What is the most common opportunistic infection in AIDS patients?

   (A) *Pneumocystis carinii* pneumonia
   (B) Toxoplasmosis
   (C) Tuberculosis

93. Petra has questions about testing her current partner. What is the appropriate time for HIV screening?

   (A) HIV testing should be done as soon as possible.
   (B) The partner should have an HIV test done at 3- and 6-month intervals from the date of unprotected sexual intercourse.
   (C) HIV testing should be done at 6-month intervals for 1 year.

Questions 94–97

Lyn complains of a sore vaginal "bump" that she first noticed 4 days ago and that has become increasingly painful. She has dysuria but no unusual vaginal discharge. Her boyfriend of 10 months had a "cold sore" on his lip and they had oral–genital relations 7 days ago. Condom use has been 70% for vaginal intercourse. Physical examination reveals temperature 99.9°F, positive inguinal nodes, and several aptheous ulcers at introitus.

94. Based on this patient's presentation, your most likely diagnosis is

   (A) Human papilloma virus (HPV)
   (B) Herpes simplex virus (HSV)
   (C) Syphilitic chancre

95. You explain to Lyn that after exposure to herpes, the incubation period is _____ days before the onset of a primary herpetic infection.

   (A) 2–7 days
   (B) 1–3 days
   (C) 7–14 days

96. The most sensitive diagnostic test for herpes is

   (A) Papanicolaou smear
   (B) Herpes culture
   (C) Serologic test for herpes

97. You provide counseling, comfort measures and education for Lyn and provide her with antiviral ointment and oral medication. You explain the oral medication will

   (A) Cure the herpes virus by reprogramming the cells' DNA
   (B) Shorten the course of the disease
   (C) Prevent recurrences

Questions 98–101

Mrs. Sohta, 30-year-old gravida 0 para 0 complains of vaginal pruritis and increased vaginal discharge. She is in day 26 of her 30-day menstrual cycle. She and her husband have been bilaterally monogamous for the last 7 years and use condoms for contraception. Her medical history is positive for adult-onset diabetes mellitus (AODM) and there is a maternal family history of gestational diabetes.

98. A predisposing factor for the development of candidal infections in this client is

   (A) Condom use
   (B) AODM
   (C) Nulliparity

99. The most common symptom of candidal infections is

   (A) Pruritis
   (B) Vaginal odor
   (C) Rash

100. Diagnosis of candidiasis is based on microscopic exam of the discharge

   (A) Mixed with normal saline
   (B) Mixed with 10% potassium hydroxide (KOH)
   (C) By Pap test

101. On wet prep you could expect to find the most common candidal species to be

(A) *Candida albicans*
(B) *Candida tropicalis*
(C) *Candida galbrata*

Questions 102–103

A 24-year-old female presents with clear, mucoid, vaginal discharge. She denies odor and has never been sexually active. She uses tampons with her menses and is currently midcycle. To determine if the leukorrhea is physiologic, you test the vaginal pH with nitrazine pH paper.

102. Normal vagina pH during the reproductive years is

(A) 3.5–4.2
(B) 5.0–5.5
(C) ≥6

103. In addition to checking the vaginal pH and wet prep, a routine test for this client would be for

(A) Gonorrhea
(B) Chlamydia
(C) Amine ("whiff" test)

Questions 104–106

Ashana, 25 years old, G0 P0, has recently returned to the United States after spending a year in Africa as part of her graduate study. She notes a mass in her groin and complains of intermittent flu-like symptoms. She admits to unprotected intercourse with a Nigerian male partner.

104. What statement is true concerning lympho-granuloma venereum (LGV)?

(A) The primary stage is characterized by multiple painless vesicular lesions with purulent discharge and associated lymphadenopathy.
(B) The secondary stage includes acute lymphadenitis with buboes.
(C) The patient initially presents with painful vulvar ulcers and bilateral inguinal lymphadenopathy.

105. The causative organism is:

(A) *Chlamydia trachomatis*
(B) *Calymmatobacterium granulomatis*
(C) *Hemophilus ducreyi*

106. The LGV titre returns as 1:64. What is the correct interpretation of this test?

(A) Negative
(B) Equivocal
(C) Positive

Questions 107–109

Ellen is an 18-year-old college student who wants you to evaluate multiple small round lesions on her genitals and thighs. She is using condoms with her new sexual partner. She admits that her boyfriend seems to have a similar rash on his thighs.

107. Molluscum contagiosum is characterized by small, firm, umbilicated papules that may be white, flesh colored, or translucent. What is the diagnostic method used to identify this lesion?

(A) Pox virus culture
(B) Tzanck culture
(C) Inspection of clinical presentation

108. What is the current treatment?

(A) No treatment as infection is self-limiting and resolves in 6–12 weeks
(B) Curette central umbilicated core and apply silver nitrate or trichloracetic acid
(C) Laser therapy

109. The clinician reviews the etiology, symptoms, transmission, and treatment with the patient. All the following statements regarding molluscum contagiosum are true EXCEPT

(A) Autoinoculation may occur in linear patterns proximal to the lesion site so the patient should be advised to avoid scratching the lesions.
(B) If the molluscum lesion becomes irritated and inflamed it may mimic a herpes lesion.
(C) Sexual contact is necessary for transmission of this virus.

Questions 110–114

A woman presents with several risk factors for a sexually transmitted infection. Her symptoms are significant for a painless vulvar lesion. Physical exam reveals one indurated ulcer on the labia majora. Inguinal nodes are negative.

110. Based on this presentation the most likely diagnosis is

    (A) Syphilitic chancre
    (B) Chancroid
    (C) Herpes genitalis

111. The causative agent of syphilis is

    (A) *Treponema pallidum*
    (B) *Hemophilus ducreyi*
    (C) *Neisseria*

112. You would expect to find secondary syphilis _____ weeks after the chancre appears; it may manifest as flu-like symptoms and lymphadenopathy.

    (A) 50–52
    (B) 4–10
    (C) 12–24

113. The major features of secondary syphilis include all of the following EXCEPT

    (A) Generalized maculopapular rash
    (B) Condylomata lata
    (C) Buboes

114. Recommended treatment for primary, or secondary, early latent (asymptomatic) syphilis of less than 1 year's duration is

    (A) Benzathine penicillin
    (B) Quinolones
    (C) Metronidazole

Questions 115–118

A married 35-year-old nulliparous woman presents with dysmenorrhea of increasing severity over the last few years and new onset dyspareunia. Menarche was at age 9; menstrual cycles are 21 days apart and last for 7 days. She is in a stable relationship and has no childbearing plans. Her family history is significant for an aunt and a sister with endometriosis. Based on her history and physical exam you suspect a possible diagnosis of endometriosis.

115. This client's risk factors for developing endometriosis are

    (A) Age
    (B) Ethnicity
    (C) Family history

116. A definitive diagnosis of endometriosis can be made by

    (A) Triad of symptoms (increased dysmenorrhea, pelvic pain, and dyspareunia) with increased CA-125
    (B) Pelvic exam
    (C) Laparoscopy

117. The goal of pharmacologic intervention in this client with endometriosis is to

    (A) Preserve future fertility
    (B) Interrupt cycles of stimulation and bleeding
    (C) Prevent endometrial cancer

118. Most recent data on the most effective treatment of endometriosis is

    (A) Tamoxifen
    (B) Gonadotropin-releasing hormone agonists (GnRH-a)
    (C) Progesterone-only minipill

Question 119

A 45-year-old multiparous woman presents with severe dysmenorrhea and menorrhagia. Bimanual exam during her menstrual period reveals a large, globular, slightly tender and softened uterus between 8 and 10 weeks in size. To rule out pelvic pathology you order an ultrasound.

119. Your working differential diagnosis includes leiomyoma, endometriosis and

    (A) Ectopic pregnancy
    (B) Adenomyosis
    (C) PID

Questions 120–125

A 46-year-old client presents with very heavy menses but is otherwise without symptoms. She denies any vasomotor symptoms associated with menopause. Her cycles are 21 days apart lasting 7 days. On physical exam you palpate a firm, irregularly shaped, enlarged uterus. You are able to outline a 6-cm mass, which is contiguous with the left lateral aspect of the fundus. The mass moves with the cervix, suggesting to you that it is likely to be a leiomyoma and not an adnexal mass.

120. In discussing her condition with her, you could advise her that fibroids (myomas, fibromyomas, and leiomyomas)

    (A) Are the most common benign tumor of the female genital tract
    (B) Are considered a premalignant tumor of the female genital tract
    (C) Usually require surgical excision with hysterectomy

121. Based on the above client's pelvic exam findings you would classify her fibroid as

    (A) Intraligamentary
    (B) Pedunculated submucosal
    (C) Pedunculated serosal

122. The most common presenting symptom of leiomyomata uteri is

    (A) Menometrorrhagia
    (B) Anemia
    (C) Dyspareunia

123. For this client with abnormal bleeding in the perimenopausal years, the appropriate management modality is

    (A) Endometrial evaluation
    (B) Pap smear
    (C) CBC with differential

124. To confirm your diagnosis of uterine fibroids in this client you would order

    (A) Ultrasound
    (B) Abdominal x-ray
    (C) Hysterosaplingogram

125. You would advise this client that leiomyomas _____ after menopause.

    (A) Progress
    (B) Regress
    (C) Remain unchanged

Questions 126–139

Annette is a 49-year-old G2 P2 who is concerned about erratic menstrual bleeding cycles. At age 45 she began to notice a shortened interval between menses from 28 days to 25 days with a lighter flow at menstruation. In the last 6 months she has had heavy to moderate bleeding every 2 weeks. She denies hot flashes but admits to feeling flushed or warm at frequent intervals during the day. Her premenstrual moods have intensified and she feels depressed for the first time in her life. She also notes a decrease in lubrication with sexual relations and occasional vulvar burning. She is a healthy non-smoking women who runs 3 miles every other day, has a low-fat diet, and works part time in retail. Her family history is significant for hypertension, and her father had a heart attack and subsequent CABG at age 68. She has one paternal aunt with breast cancer diagnosed at age 79. She has no family history of osteoporosis.

126. What mechanism is thought to be responsible for the initial shortening of the interval between menstrual bleeding?

    (A) Anovulation
    (B) decrease in serum estradiol
    (C) decrease in serum progesterone

127. Genitourinary atrophy occurs rapidly in the absence of sufficient estrogen. Epithelial tissues that show atrophic changes with symptoms of dryness, thinness, and resulting dyspareunia, as well as evidence of mucosal changes suggesting deficiency on clinical exam can be restored with estrogen therapy. How long will it take to restore these tissues in this patient's situation?

    (A) Estrogen-replacement therapy (ERT) can restore affected tissue in 6–8 weeks.
    (B) When the underlying dermis is affected, clinical improvement and symptomatic relief may take 12–24 months.
    (C) Complete reversal of symptoms may not be possible without a lifelong commitment to ERT.

128. Nearly 50% of menopausal women complain of sudden sensations of flushing and extreme warmth followed by profuse sweating. Identify the correct statement associated with hot flashes.

(A) Hot flashes precede LH and FSH rises by just a few minutes.
(B) Hot flashes occur following complete cessation of menses.
(C) Vasomotor stability reverses itself within 1 year after cessation of menses.

129. Estrogen deprivation may cause which of the following?

(A) Contraction of pelvic ligaments and muscles
(B) Decreased glycogen production leading to a more alkaline pH of the vagina
(C) Increased adipose tissue of the breast

130. Osteoporosis risk is associated with estrogen deprivation. Identify other factors that may be implicated in increased risk.

(A) Positive family history
(B) African-American background
(C) Low-protein diet

131. DEXA (dual x-ray photon absorptiometry) has become accepted as the diagnostic method for identifying postmenopausal women at risk for osteoporotic fractures. What are the most reliable measurements that can be taken as predictors of osteoporosis risk?

(A) Vertebral bodies
(B) Wrist–distal radius
(C) Spine and hip

132. When one reviews the results of the DEXA scan, what is the most reliable measurement of actual risk and need for therapy?

(A) Age-corrected average
(B) Peak bone mass 1 standard deviation above the mean
(C) Peak bone mass 2.5 standard deviations below the mean

133. What preventive measures should be discussed with perimenopausal women?

(A) Swimming at least three times per week
(B) Increasing calcium intake to 1500 mg per day
(C) Adding protein-rich food to diet

134. What dose of ERT is needed to impact on bone mass?

(A) Estradiol 1 mg po daily
(B) Premarin 0.625 mg po daily
(C) Premarin 0.325 mg po daily

135. During the first 5 years following menopause, calcium loss occurs primarily from which type of bone?

(A) Vertebral
(B) Hip
(C) Long bones

136. The rates of myocardial infarction, angina, and sudden cardiac death increase in women during the sixth through eighth decades of life to become equal to or slightly greater than those of age-matched men, suggesting that premenopausal estrogen levels may be a protective factor. It is well established that plasma lipoprotein patterns predict risk of coronary artery disease. What lipoprotein fraction is most dependent on or influenced by estrogen?

(A) HDL
(B) LDL
(C) Total cholesterol

137. ERT has a significant cardioprotective effect. The PEPI study concluded that estrogen has an impact on improved health in several ways. Choose one way estrogen exerts its positive impact.

(A) Increased fibrinogen levels
(B) Inhibition of deposition of LDL on artery walls
(C) Decrease in vasomotor tone

138. Endometrial cancer is a significant risk for women taking unopposed estrogen. Adding progesterone can reduce this risk. What management steps must be included before this patient can be considered for HRT?

(A) Measurements of serum FSH and LH and an endometrial biopsy
(B) Measurements of FSH and LH and a transvaginal ultrasound
(C) Measurements of FSH and LH only

139. Breast cancer is a major concern for all women and a significant factor to consider prior to placing women on ERT. What recent findings reflect the current status of breast cancer and ERT?

(A) The Nurses Health Study found no association between breast cancer and ERT.
(B) Women currently on ERT for 5–9 years have a relative risk of 1.5 compared to women who never used ERT.
(C) Death rates from breast cancer in ERT users exceed the rates of sudden death from cardiovascular disease in women who elect not to use ERT.

Questions 140–142

Mary, a 60-year-old G0 P0, has an appointment for her annual examination. The patient says she is in good health without chronic illness or use of regular medications. The clinician questions her about any changes in bladder or bowel habits and she admits to abdominal bloating, increased gas and constipation, and a low backache. She denies dysuria, frequency, and burning but does note occasional bladder pressure. Her last menses was at age 51 years and she did not elect to take hormones as her menopausal symptoms were minimal.

140. The clinician reviews Mary's history to identify risk factors for ovarian cancer. Which risk is the most significant?

(A) Lynch II syndrome (Cancer Family Syndrome)
(B) Maternal aunt with a history of ovarian cancer
(C) Nulliparity

141. The clinician palpates a right adnexal mass measuring 1.0   2.0   3.0 cm. The mass is firm, solid and nontender. The uterus is small and regular. The left ovary is not palpable. What is the next step in management?

(A) Reassure the patient that the right ovary is normal in size and educate the patient about dietary and lifestyle changes that will improve bowel function.
(B) Perform transvaginal ultrasound.
(C) Draw blood for CA-125 biologic tumor marker.

142. Mary has surgery and is diagnosed with a stage II epithelial tumor. Her follow-up care will include chemotherapy followed by an interval history, pelvic examination, and CA-125 every 2–3 months for 2 years. What is true about the CA-125 tumor marker?

(A) An elevated CA-125 following surgery and chemotherapy may indicate relapse.
(B) CA-125 is considered sensitive and specific enough to be used as a screen for ovarian cancer in the general population.
(C) CA-125 levels decrease during menses.

Questions 143–147

Somalia is a 55-year-old G2 P2 who presents at the office for evaluation of the sudden onset of vaginal bleeding. Her last menstrual period was 2 years ago. At that time her FSH level was 45 mIU/mL. She declined starting hormone replacement therapy at that time although she did use Premarin cream for 12 months because of dyspareunia. She did not take progesterone during that year. She describes the bleeding as heavy with clots. She is using one maxi-pad per hour and the volume seems to be increasing. She denies fever or chills but admits to low back pain and cramping.

143. What is the greatest risk factor of endometrial cancer?

(A) Diabetes
(B) Hypertension
(C) Unopposed estrogen use

144. What risk is not associated with endometrial cancer?

(A) Obesity
(B) Polycystic ovarian disease
(C) Oral contraceptive use

145. Evaluation of postmenopausal vaginal bleeding must rule out cancer. What procedure would you choose to rule out cancer in this patient?

(A) Hysteroscopy
(B) Dilatation and curettage
(C) Endometrial biopsy

146. Somalia is diagnosed with stage 1B endometrial cancer. This stage is defined as

(A) Localized to the endometrium
(B) Endometrium with invasion to less than half of the myometrium
(C) Endometrium and endocervical involvement

147. What is the treatment of stage 1A endometrial cancer in a patient with no other risks?

(A) Total abdominal hysterectomy and bilateral oophorectomy
(B) Total abdominal hysterectomy and bilateral oophorectomy plus radiation
(C) Chemotherapy and radiation

Questions 148–150

Dinah is a 46-year-old G3 P3 who presents at the office complaining of a 21-day episode of vaginal bleeding. The onset occurred at the expected time of her menses but is heavier in flow with clots and cramping. Her prior 6 menstrual cycles have been irregular in interval but lasting only 3–4 days. She denies chronic illness and does not take any regular medications. She uses a diaphragm for contraception. Her last Pap smear and gynecologic exam were 1 year ago.

148. What is the most significant historical information the clinician must elicit?

(A) Symptoms of thyroid disease
(B) Changes in menstrual flow and pattern as compared to normal pattern and associated symptoms
(C) Daily menstrual pad or tampon count

149. A diagnosis of dysfunctional uterine bleeding has been made. This diagnosis is commonly associated with which of the following in the perimenopausal woman?

(A) Uterine fibroids
(B) Cervical polyps
(C) Disruption in the cyclic release of GnRH, FSH, or LH

150. What diagnostic procedure must be considered in Dinah's evaluation?

(A) Transvaginal ultrasound
(B) Endometrial biopsy
(C) Diagnostic dilatation and curettage

Questions 151–154

A 19-year-old African-American woman presents with a nontender, unilateral breast lump in the right breast, which she noticed on breast self-exam. Her last menstrual period was normal and ended 2 days ago. She denies pain, nipple discharge, or recent trauma.

151. The most likely diagnosis is fibrocystic breast changes versus

(A) Fibroadenoma
(B) Breast cancer
(C) Fat necrosis

152. You would expect the above client to be at which of Tanner's stages for breast development?

(A) Stage 3
(B) Stage 4
(C) Stage 5

153. Based on your working diagnosis, which diagnostic test would you select initially?

(A) Ultrasound
(B) Mammogram
(C) Thermography

154. Which is the most definitive diagnostic method you could order for this young woman?

(A) Ultrasound
(B) Mammogram
(C) Fine-needle aspiration (FNA)

Questions 155–156

A 32-year-old woman complains of long-standing, scattered, tender, pea-sized breast "lumps" and one new slightly larger lump in the upper outer region of the right breast. She is on Ovcon 35. Her family and personal history are negative for breast cancer. She is in day 19 of her OC cycle.

155.   Your most likely diagnosis would be

(A) Fibrocystic breast changes
(B) Breast cancer
(C) Nonpuerperal mastitis

156.   Women with fibrocystic breast disease (FBD) usually present with

(A) No relationship of breast symptoms to menstrual cycle
(B) Breast symptoms that may change according to the stage of the menstrual period
(C) Breast exam that involves axillary lymphadenopathy

Questions 157–158

A 45-year-old white female presents with fibrocystic breast changes but no dominant breast lump. She is a gravida 1 para 1 with age at first pregnancy 27 years. Her last menstrual period was 2 weeks ago and normal. Her history is significant for a mother and two sisters with fibrocystic nodularity. Her caffeine intake includes 2 to 3 cups of coffee daily and an occasional cola or tea. She takes no nonprescription medications. She does not smoke. Menarche was at age 12.

157.   What is her most significant risk factor for breast cancer?

(A) History of FBD
(B) Family history of FBD
(C) Age

158.   The most sensitive method for detection of breast cancer in the above client would be

(A) Diagnostic mammography
(B) Ultrasound
(C) Screening mammogram

Questions 159–160

Mrs. Simon, a 34-year-old multiparous female, recently discontinued breastfeeding her 14-month-old daughter. She complains of persistent yellowish-white nipple discharge and a painless lump located near the nipple.

159.   The most likely diagnosis is:

(A) Puerperal mastitis
(B) Galactocele
(C) Intraductal papilloma

160.   With the client presenting with galactorrhea you would order

(A) Prolactin
(B) CBC with differential
(C) BRCA1

Question 161

161.   According the American Cancer Society, women over 50 should be screened with a mammogram

(A) Yearly
(B) Every two years
(C) Left to the discretion of the individual provider

Questions 162–163

A 17-year-old high school junior comes to the office complaining of painful menstrual cramps on the first 2 days of her menses since age 14. The pain is colicky in nature, located in the suprapubic area. She has tried Tylenol with some effect. Menarche was at 13 years with normal development of secondary sex characteristics. The client has never been sexually active.

162.   In this client you would distinguish between primary and secondary dysmenorrhea based on

(A) The nature of the pain
(B) Absence of pelvic pathology
(C) The location of the pain

163. The pharmacologic treatment of choice this client would be

    (A) Oral contraceptives
    (B) Nonsteroidal antiinflammatory (NSAIDs)
    (C) Aspirin

Questions 164–168

Dora is a 35-year-old G1 P1 who complains of urinary frequency, urgency, and bladder pain. Her major complaint is the need to urinate every 20 minutes. This is very disruptive during the day and night. She denies fever, chills, or back pain. She notes vaginal discharge without odor, pruritus, or dyspareunia. She denies sexually transmitted disease risk, although last intercourse did occur directly before the onset of symptoms. She has a history of prior UTIs and has had an appointment with a urologist for evaluation of urinary frequency and pain that often persists despite treatment. He has discussed the possibility of cystoscopic evaluation to rule out interstitial cystitis.

164. The clinician orders a urinalysis and urine culture. The urinalysis is negative for blood, nitrites, and leukocytes. The pH is 5.0 with a specific gravity of 1010. The urine culture is sent out to the lab. What results would you expect to see in a patient with interstitial cystitis?

    (A) Urine culture > 100,000 *E. coli* organisms
    (B) Urine culture: no growth
    (C) Urine culture > 10,000 enterococci

165. All the criteria following diagnose interstitial cystitis EXCEPT

    (A) Frequent nocturia
    (B) Urinary frequency of greater than eight times during waking hours
    (C) Symptoms relieved by antibiotics

166. What characteristics are *not* associated with interstitial cystitis?

    (A) Hunner's ulcer can be identified by cystoscopy.
    (B) Bladder capacity is < 300 mL on cystometry in patients who are awake.
    (C) Symptoms have a gradual onset and increase in intensity over several years.

167. You review Dora's cystoscopic findings. What in the report will help to diagnose her syndrome as interstitial cystitis?

    (A) Glomerulations of the bladder wall
    (B) Bladder calculi
    (C) Normal findings

168. What treatment option might be considered for this patient if diagnosed with interstitial cystitis?

    (A) Long-term course of broad-spectrum antibiotics
    (B) Hydraulic distention and instillation of dimethyl sulfoxide (DMSO)
    (C) Prophylactic antispasmodic drug use such as Pyridium

Questions 169–171

Jerri presents with complaints of intermittent pelvic pain of 2 weeks' duration. This acute episode is similar to prior pain episodes over the last several years. She is a 28-year-old G0 P0 with a history of dysmenorrhea since menarche and Progestasert IUD use at age 23 that resulted in PID. She is currently in a long-term monogamous relationship and uses condoms for birth control. Her last normal menstrual period was 4 weeks ago. She denies fever, chills, abnormal discharge, or dysuria. She admits to dyspareunia and pain with bowel movements. She noted slight spotting following her last intercourse. She is currently being evaluated for chronic fatigue and constipation by her primary care clinician.

169. Pelvic pain that is intermittent but of several years' duration may have multiple etiologies. Which must be be included as a first step in evaluating this patient?

    (A) Rule out ectopic pregnancy
    (B) Laparoscopic evaluation to rule out pelvic adhesions
    (C) Review of nutrition and bowel habits to evaluate patient for irritable bowel syndrome

170. All the following are commonly associated with chronic pelvic pain EXCEPT

(A) Irritable bowel syndrome
(B) Recurrent vaginitis
(C) Endometriosis

171. Which statement is true about laparoscopy?

(A) Positive laparoscopic findings and pathology can predict pain level.
(B) Laparoscopic findings that are negative can assure a woman that she is normal.
(C) Laparoscopy can diagnose endometriosis and adhesions and biopsy suspicious areas.

Questions 172–177

Jana is a 25-year-old woman who has an appointment for her annual examination and Pap smear. The patient had a gynecologic evaluation 3 years prior, which resulted in an incomplete examination without speculum or bimanual exam. History reveals a healthy G0 P0 with no allergies, medication use, or chronic illness or history of hospitalizations. Patient denies known history of sexual abuse. Patient sees a psychotherapist at weekly intervals for anxiety and recurrent nightmares. Jana has normal menstrual cycles with menarche at age 13 years. She denies vaginal discharge, odor, pruritis, and dysuria. She does not use tampons regularly nor has ever had a sexual relationship. She denies masturbation or orgasm and admits to feelings of nausea when touching the genital area. At the present time Jana has started a platonic relationship that she hopes will develop into something more intimate.

172. All the statements regarding vaginismus are correct EXCEPT

(A) Involves involuntary spasmodic contractions of the pubococcygeus muscles, introitus, and outer third of the vagina
(B) Is not associated with sexual trauma
(C) Can often be managed easily once the underlying infectious cause is identified and treated

173. What is the current treatment of vaginismus?

(A) Low-dose tricyclic antidepressant therapy
(B) Behavior modification using dilators in graduated sizes for self-insertion
(C) Vestibular surgery

174. The evaluation of Jana should include a sexual history. Jana admits to feelings of arousal, sexual dreams, and vaginal lubrication with arousal, but has been unable to engage in genital touch by herself or with a partner. Which category of sexual dysfunction would be considered in Jana's assessment? Choose more than one answer if applicable:

(A) Inhibited sexual desire
(B) Anorgasmia
(C) Sexual aversion disorder

175. Anorgasmia may be defined as

(A) Inability to experience desire and arousal with partner
(B) Absence of orgasm by individual following sufficient stimulation
(C) Uncontrollable introital spasmodic contractions associated with attempts at penetration

176. Jana denies any history of masturbation and orgasm. What might be included in her initial management plan?

(A) Clinician identification of normal anatomy and physiology of genitalia and identification of genital organs using diagrams and a patient-held mirror during pelvic examination; instructing patient in relaxation breathing and genital touch
(B) Instructions to the couple regarding mutual genital touch
(C) Partner exploration and participation of manual stimulation in a relaxed setting

177. Researchers have identified four stages of sexual response. Choose the true statement.

(A) Men and women experience similar sexual responses in four stages: excitement, plateau, orgasm, and resolution.
(B) Men and women have a refractory period that follows orgasm where they are unable to achieve a subsequent orgasm.
(C) The plateau stage of muscle tension, tissue engorgement, elevated heart and respiratory rates, and increased blood pressure lasts for several seconds and resolves.

Questions 178–180

Rosa presents at your office as a new patient. You review her medical history form and note that she has answered affirmatively to history of rape but has not included the date of the incident. She lists the reason for her visit as one to treat a persistent vaginal discharge. She also lists inability to sleep and confusion as two other health concerns.

178. The clinician questions Rosa about the rape occurrence and the patient admits that it occurred at 11 o'clock last night. The patient is tearful but declines the offer of reporting the rape. What is the next step in clinical evaluation?

   (A) Urge the patient to report the rape occurrence and call the police so that the patient may discuss this option with an officer.
   (B) Conduct a physical exam and collect forensic samples including pubic hair, scrapings, vaginal sampling, and culture for sexually transmitted diseases.
   (C) Treat prophylactically for pregnancy and common STDs.

179. Rape Trauma Syndrome (RTS) is classified as a posttraumatic stress disorder in the *Diagnostic and Statistical Manual of Mental Disorders*. Which statement is true concerning RTS?

   (A) Research studies show that acquaintance rapes are easier to resolve.
   (B) When women are evaluated several years post assault, those who experienced rape are more likely to receive a diagnosis of major depression, generalized anxiety, or obsessive compulsive disorders when compared to the women who have not been raped.
   (C) The acute phase of the Rape Trauma Syndrome occurs immediately after the assault or after disclosing the assault. Symptoms include tearfulness, agitation, or calmness. This initial stage lasts 24 hours.

180. The history of the assault must include relevant social and gynecologic information. Which part of the patient's history is not directly relevant to the rape assessment?

   (A) Did the patient shower, douche, or bathe during the hours following the event?
   (B) What are current relationship status, last intercourse, and contraception used?
   (C) Did the patient resist the attack by the perpetrator?

Questions 181–186

An 35-year-old Hispanic female presents with oligomenorrhea, hirsutism, oily skin, and acne. She denies voice changes or hoarseness.

181. What is your most likely diagnosis?

   (A) Depression
   (B) Rheumatoid arthritis
   (C) Polycystic ovarian syndrome (PCO)

182. A key feature of PCO is

   (A) Anovulation
   (B) Obesity
   (C) Alopecia and acne

183. The primary factor in hirsutism is

   (A) An increase in androgen levels
   (B) Decreased TSH
   (C) Decreased estradiol levels

184. Because this client has PCO, you would expect her hormonal levels to be as follows:

   (A) LH levels elevated; FSH levels low or normal
   (B) LH low or normal; FSH high or normal
   (C) FSH and LH normal

185. The effect of unopposed and uninterrupted estrogen in the amenorrheic woman can put her at considerable risk for

   (A) Breast cancer before age 45
   (B) Endometrial cancer
   (C) Osteoporosis

186. Endometrial biopsy should be considered as part of the workup based on

(A) Amount of DUB
(B) Duration of exposure to unopposed estrogen
(C) Patient's age

Question 187

A young woman presents with a history of having had only two menstrual periods during the last 12 months. LMP was 4 months ago. You review her history carefully. She denies stress or anxiety, anorexia nervosa, acute weight loss, or crash dieting. You rule out pregnancy.

187. The next step in her workup would be

(A) TSH level
(B) Hysterosalpingogram
(C) CT scan of the sella turcica

Answers and Rationales for Gynecology Cases

1. **(A)** The etiology of Premenstrual Syndrome (PMS) is unknown but is considered a complex disorder linked to the cyclic activity of the hypothalamic–pituitary–ovarian axis with interactions between ovarian steroid hormones, endogenous opioid peptides, central neurotransmitters, prostaglandins, and the autonomic and endocrine systems. Nutrition as well as endocrine and lifestyle factors have a role in symptomatology. The incidence is estimated at 20–80% in reproductive age women. At the current time the syndrome is poorly understood and treatments are targeted at reducing or relieving individual symptoms. Clients present with a number of physical and emotional symptoms that interfere with optimal functioning during the luteal phase of the menstrual cycle and are relieved at the onset of bleeding. Appropriate diagnosis requires documentation of the cyclicity of symptoms. Between 25 and 75% of all women presumed to have PMS will be found to have another medical condition such as hypothyroidism, Cushing Syndrome, noncyclical anxiety, or severe psychosis. Women who have undergone hysterectomy with ovaries left intact may still experience PMS. The timing of the follicular and luteal phase may require measurement of circulating reproductive hormones to make the correct diagnosis.

2. **(C)** The patient requires a comprehensive history, physical examination, and lab tests to rule out other medical conditions that could be causing or exacerbating the symptom complex. Differential diagnosis should be considered for the specific symptoms or cluster of symptoms. There are no uniform criteria for PMS diagnosis nor standard laboratory guidelines. It is advisable to perform thyroid function tests as hypothyroidism is frequently encountered and underdiagnosed in these patients. Such tests as prolactin, CBC, FSH and LH, and glucose may be considered but are likely to have a low yield in a general clinic setting. The most common error in the management of PMS is reliance on retrospective data from previous clinic visits. More than 150 symptoms have been associated with PMS and although the symptom complex is important, it is the repeated cyclical clustering of symptoms that confirms the diagnosis. The patient should keep a daily diary of symptoms for at least 2–3 cycles. This should be reviewed by the patient and clinician.

3. **(A)** Dietary changes are one of the initial measures in management. It is advised to increase the intake of complex carbohydrates and decrease salt, refined sugar and caffeine during the luteal phase. Premenstrual weight gain may be a normal occurrence caused by salt and water retention although PMS patients do not have consistent weight changes and there is no correlation between weight gain and other symptoms. Women who exercise regularly report fewer premenstrual symptoms than nonathletic women. Exercise may stimulate serotoninergic activity although this is hypothesized as it is not known why exercise decreases symptoms. Progesterone withdrawal or deficiency may be associated with PMS as progesterone levels decrease during the luteal phase. Randomized double-blind studies fail to show that progesterone is significantly more effective than placebo despite higher circulating progesterone levels. Women do seem to report improvement of symptoms when the progesterone is used as one of the treatment

options. Prozac is considered an appropriate alternative when initial self-care regimens are ineffective.

4. **(C)** Nutritional counseling should stress a high-complex-carbohydrate, low-fat diet. Christiane Northrup notes that nutritional characteristics of women with PMS include high consumption of dairy, refined sugar, and animal fat with deficiencies in vitamins C and E, selenium, and magnesium. Many woman admit to symptomatic relief with diet modification and vitamin supplementation that includes magnesium, B complex, evening primrose oil and antioxidants. Acupuncture also helps to relieve many of the symptoms. Vitamin E may alleviate breast symptoms. The patient should be instructed not to exceed a dose of 800 IU because excessive vitamin E can increase her bleeding time. Scientific studies of vitamin use in alleviation of PMS remain inconclusive.

5. **(B)** Loestrin 1/20 Fe either 21-day OCs with 21 days of active hormone of the same dose or 28-day with 21 days of hormone and 7 days of a placebo or sugar pill. Loestrin is the only OC that provides 50 mg of iron in the placebo pills for the week off the hormone.

    All women who take OCs should take the lowest possible dose formulation that is effective. Low-dose norethindrone, which slightly elevates HDL-2 cholesterol, may be prescribed as Modicon, Brevicon, or Ovcon. The fourth-generation progestin norgestimate (Ortho-Cylcen and Ortho-TriCylcen) would also be a good choice.

    When starting OCs a *good rule of thumb* is to begin with an OC that contains 35 µg or less of estrogen in the form of ethinyl estradiol (EE) and the equivalent of 0.4 or 0.5 mg norethindrone. OCs with estrogen doses above 35 µg may increase the incidence of thromboembolic disease. Ovral is an OC with a 50 µg EE dose and the most potent form of progesterone with levonorgestrel.

    It should be noted that teens' biggest concerns are weight gain and acne. Patients' acne will improve because OCs lower testosterone levels and OCs do not cause weight gain.

6. **(A)** Patients who have a family history of heart disease should have a cardiac profile, which includes a fasting cholesterol screen (including total, HDL, and LDL) and triglycerides. Since the patient has a family history of diabetes, a fasting blood sugar should be obtained before starting OCs. Physical exam needs to include blood pressure and thyroid, cardiac, respiratory, breast, pelvic, and abdominal exam (to check for hepatosplenomegaly or masses), extremities, and Pap smear, all of which should be normal.

    Low dose OCs do not produce a diabetic glucose tolerance response and there is no evidence that OCs increase the incidence of DM. FBS should be checked annually. Liver function tests (alkaline phosphatase and transaminase) are not routinely recommended for screening purposes for clients on OCs. It should be noted that *absolute* contraindications to OCs are hepatic ademonas, carcinoma, or benign liver tumors. Steroid components of OCs differ from the natural sex steroid produced in the ovaries because OCs enter the hepatic circulation via the gastrointestinal (GI) tract and portal vein. The body's natural ovarian hormones enter the systemic circulation via ovarian veins and the inferior vena cava, thereby bypassing the liver. Steroid hormones may be poorly metabolized in women with impaired liver function.

    OCs are not contraindicated in this client. She is at very low risk since she is under 35 years of age and a nonsmoker.

7. **(A)** No backup contraceptive method is needed if the OCs are begun on the first day of menses since ovulation is inhibited for that cycle. The pill works primarily by suppressing ovulation (via suppressing release of gonadotropin-releasing hormone [GnRH], which inhibits the pituitary release of FSH and LH), causing thick cervical mucus (which makes it difficult for sperm to penetrate) and making endometrium or lining of the uterus unfavorable for implantation.

    Sunday start is the second best answer. If menses begin on a Monday the OCs would not be started until 6 days or the following Sunday. Thus, a second backup method of contraception would be needed the first 7 days after beginning the OCs (or the first full week on the OCs). Prevention of ovulation may not occur if OCs are started after the fifth menstrual day.

As a general rule, a second method of contraception should always be prescribed when dispensing OCs. Also remember OCs provide no STD protection, so give Rx with condom samples.

8. **(A)** Provide support and reassurance, because breakthrough bleeding (BTB) or spotting is always greatest during the first few cycles of OC use as the endometrium or uterine lining is adjusting to lower amounts of estrogen and progesterone without OCs. BTB decreases between the second and fourth cycles and then plateaus off. BTB is the most common reason women discontinue OCs, so provide additional supportive reassurance that the problem usually resolves by 3 months, that the pill is still working, and that it is not medically dangerous.

Endometrial activity of an OC is measured best by how well the OC prevents breakthrough bleeding or spotting.

9. **(A)** Menses will be lighter, because the pill decreases the amount of menstrual blood (which will provide an improvement in her hemoglobin). Menses will be regular and dysmenorrhea will improve on OCs. Menstrual pain that has been resistant to treatment with prostaglandin inhibitors such as Motrin, Advil, Anaprox, or Ponstel may respond more favorably to OCs.

10. **(A)** Dysfunctional uterine bleeding (DUB) in adolescents is most often due to immaturity of the hypothalamic–pituitary unit or the polycystic ovarian syndrome. Studies have shown that anovulation results from an absence of a cyclic surge of gonadotropins. In some cases this is the result of the inability of the hypothalamic-pituitary axis to respond to increases in estradiol. Anovulation in adolescents with polycystic ovary syndrome is often associated with elevation of pituitary LH and secretion of ovarian estrogens and androgens. There is an absence of a cyclic surge of gonadotropins, which is the result of a persistent elevation of ovarian estrogens and/or androgens. Dysfunctional or anovulatory bleeding is the result of the effects of unopposed estrogen on the uterine endometrium. In the absence of progesterone, the endometrium becomes thicker and extremely vascular, but fragile owing to lack of structural support from progesterone. As a result, spontaneous and unpredictable bleeding occurs randomly throughout the endometrium. In addition, the endometrial vessels do not constrict to limit the duration and extent of bleeding.

11. **(A)** Chronic illness such as hypothyroidism, AIDS, coagulation defects, massive obesity, kidney and liver disease, and cancer can impact on the hypothalamic–pituitary axis. Drugs such as steroids, phenothiazides, digitalis, amphetamines, and anticholinergics can also effect ovulatory status. Stress has been identified as a precipitating event associated with anovulation and subsequent DUB. It is very important to include assessment of stress levels in the history. Other factors that may precipitate DUB are diet change, weight gain or loss, sleep loss, mental strain, and alcohol or illicit drug use. Excessive athletic activity or exercise is associated with anovulatory cycles and can result in temporary menstrual cessation and/or dysfunctional uterine bleeding. Exercise patterns and weight and height should be documented.

12. **(B)** Dysfunctional uterine bleeding in the adolescent is associated with an absence of consistent surges of FSH and LH due to immaturity of the hypothalamic–pituitary–ovarian (HPO) axis at early onset of menarche. Often the typical profile following the onset of menarche is an absence of regular menses for 1–12 cycles followed by an unpredictable uterine bleeding episode that may last longer than the expected length of a bleeding cycle. This is the result of the buildup of unopposed estrogen. Complete irregular bleeding caused by unopposed estrogen may result in metrorrhagia (episodes of vaginal bleeding between normal bleeding cycles), menorrhagia (bleeding occurring at the regular interval but the volume of blood loss is greater and the duration may be extended by only a few days), or menometrorrhagia (indicates both increased blood volume loss and bleeding beyond the expected duration). Premenstrual

molimina and dysmenorrhea are not commonly associated with anovulatory bleeding cycles. The clinician may direct questions appropriate to the assessment of ovulatory status. This may include the following: evidence of mittelschmerz, increased midcycle mucus, premenstrual molimina, dysmenorrhea, and a biphasic basal body temperature pattern (at the time of ovulation, the temperature usually rises 1°F and remains elevated until the onset of bleeding).

13. **(A)** This syndrome is the result of a combination of androgen excess and anovulation. LH levels are elevated and FSH levels are low normal. Increased androgens result in elevated estradiol levels, which further decrease FSH. Alterations of hormone levels interfere with GnRH secretion and follicular development. Excess androgen levels may result in hirsutism, clitoral enlargement, voice changes, and increased muscle mass. Polycystic ovarian disease (PCOD) is associated with hyperandrogenism, insulin resistance, and acanthosis nigricans in women. Familial clustering of PCOD with autosomal dominance has also been demonstrated. Adolescents with PCOD often have oligomenorrhea where the sustained elevation of LH and secretion of androgens and estrogen by the ovary prevents a consistent cyclic surge and ovulation does not occur.

14. **(A)** A speculum and bimanual examination must be included in the evaluation of the adolescent with abnormal vaginal bleeding. Inspection of the vagina may reveal a laceration, lesion, or tampon-induced ulcer. Cervical lesions rarely result in bleeding in this age group, but the clinician must rule out cervical lesions or polyps. Cyanosis of the cervix may be associated with intrauterine pregnancy, which must always be included in the differential diagnosis. Ectopic pregnancy must also be considered and a routine pregnancy test ordered regardless of history of sexual activity. A complete blood count and differential should be ordered to assess for evidence of anemia and platelet disorders. Pelvic ultrasound is not considered routine in initial management of the adolescent with DUB, but if findings on routine pelvic examination indicate an adnexal mass or uterine enlargement, an ultrasound may be indicated. Transvaginal ultrasound has the advantage of evaluating the endometrium for thickness and evidence of lesions. This is an indirect assessment of endometrial activity. A positive pregnancy test would also indicate a need for pelvic ultrasound.

15. **(A)** Depo-Provera injections inhibit ovulation by suppression of FSH and LH. The circulating level of progestin is high enough to block the LH surge. FSH is not completely blocked and continues to produce estrogen. Depo-Provera impacts on the endometrium and cervical mucus. The endometrium becomes shallow and atrophic and the cervical mucus thick and hostile to sperm. Follicular growth is sufficent to produce estrogen levels comparable to those in the follicular phase of a normal menstrual cycle thereby preventing symptoms of estrogen deficiency.

16. **(A)** Depo-Provera can be considered for patients with congenital heart disease, sickle cell anemia, or a previous history of thromboembolism. Women over 35 years of age who smoke are also candidates for this contraceptive. The absolute safety in regard to thrombosis is mainly theoretical, without research studies. No increase in thrombosis has been noted in Depo-Provera users.

Decreased bone density has been reported in one retrospective study of 30 women. The findings were reversible upon discontinuation of use. The criticism of the study is that no baseline bone density measurements were taken prior to Depo-Provera use. Future research will be addressing the risk of osteoporosis in Depo-Provera users.

17. **(A)** Depo-Provera 150 mg/mL is injected as an aqueous suspension of microcrystals deep in the gluteal or deltoid muscle. The low solubility of the microcrystals at the injection site results in prolonged circulating levels of the active progestogen. The levels remain elevated for 3–4 months. The ideal time to initiate Depo-Provera is within 5 days of the onset of normal menses in order to inhibit ovulation. The typical failure rate associated with Depo-Provera use is 0.3%, comparable to tubal ligation and Norplant.

18. **(C)** Discussion of the use, side effects, and risks of contraceptive options should be discussed in detail prior to dispensing the particular method. A written consent form should be reviewed and signed by the patient and witnessed by the clinician. This document should be part of the clinical record and updated annually. Counseling about sexually transmitted–disease risk is an important component of management when the contraceptive chosen is not protective against these infections. Adjunctive barrier methods and assessment of individual partner risk should be discussed prior to injection. Resolving the status of past abnormal Pap results are important but not essential prior to Depo-Provera injection.

19. **(A)** Depo-Provera should be given every 12 weeks to ensure optimal pregnancy protection. The injection can be given up to 14 weeks following the last dose. The goal of management in this case is to rule out pregnancy prior to injection. Probabilty of pregnancy requires knowledge of last intercourse, bleeding patterns, and dates of the last few bleeding episodes to assess ovulatory status. This patient denies intercourse for 2 months. In this case a urine pregnancy test would be adequate to rule out pregnancy. Advise the patient to use condoms and foam for the first 2 weeks following injection.

20. **(C)** Repeated urinary tract infection (UTIs; cystitis) secondary to compression and irritation of the urethra. A diaphragm that is too large may also be a factor in recurrent UTIs. Other contraindications are inability to achieve satisfactory fit, allergy to rubber or spermicide (rare), and chronic constipation (can cause discomfort).

Neither pelvic relaxation nor irregular menstrual cycles (ie; anovulatory cycles) are contraindications to diaphragm use.

21. **(C)** The arching-spring rim diaphragm has a very sturdy, firm rim. It can be used despite pelvic relaxation even with a cystocele (bulging of the bladder into the vagina) and/or a rectocele (rectal hernia bulging into the posterior vagina, usually resulting from childbirth) or lax vaginal muscle tone. Reinforce the need to wait

at least 6 hours after intercourse before removing the diaphragm or douching.

The flat-spring rim has a soft, gentle rim and is a good choice for the nulliparous woman or those with a shallow notch behind the pubic bone. It folds flat for insertion.

The coil spring has a sturdy rim and is good for women with average muscle tone and average pubic arch notch.

The wide-seal rim has a flexible flange attached to the inner rim, which is intended to hold the spermicide and create a better seal between the diaphragm and the vaginal wall. Available in both coil-spring and arching-spring rim types.

22. **(B)** Simple effective emergency options are available and using them is legal (though not FDA approved). Diaphragms require that the user remain highly motivated; they can also become dislodged. Though the chance of pregnancy with unprotected intercourse in one cycle is low patients should be aware of this Rx. Postcoital hormonal contraception is most effective if given within the first 12–24 hours after unprotected intercourse and is considered ineffective if after 72 hours. The usual procedure is to take two low-dose OCs 12 hours apart (total 200 g ethinyl estradiol and 2 mg of norgestrel or 1 mg of levonorgestrel [2 Ovral or 4 Lo/Ovral, Nordette, or Levlen 12 hours apart; or Triphasil or Tri-Levlen (yellow pills only) 12 hours apart]). Giving low-dose OCs within 72 hours creates an inadequate or absent luteal phase. Thus, the endometrium is out of phase and implantation will be unfavorable. There may also be interference with fertilization and disordered tubal transport.

IUD insertion (up to 7 days after ovulation, when intercourse has occurred earlier in the cycle) and danazol are options for women who cannot use estrogen.

Barriers with spermicide provide protection against STD consequences such as PID and give the best protection against cervical neoplasia. In this client this is not a concern since she is monogamous and at low risk for STDs.

23. **(A)** LAM is a highly effective, temporary method of contraception provided the following criteria are adhered to: another method

of contraception is used when the lactating woman resumes menstruation, bottle feeds are introduced, or at 6 months. In order to rely on LAM as a temporary method of birth control, lactating women must avoid any bottle feedings and provide only minimal supplements by spoon or cup. Lactating women who provide bottle supplements need to use another method of birth control no later than their first 6-week postpartum exam.

24. (C) Informed consent is the basis of contraception decision making. Prior to IUD insertion this client would need to be counseled regarding condom use and STD/HIV risk factors. She would need to be screened for all the STDs prior to IUD insertion.

Ideal candidates for the IUD are women in a monogamous relationship who want reversible, safe, long-acting contraception (such as women who have completed their families but do not want a tubal sterilization or cannot take OCs). Use of an IUD by women with one sexual partner does not increase their rate of infection or tubal infertility. Populations at greatest risk for IUD complications are women with multiple sexual partners, history of PID, nulliparous, and under 25 years old. The IUD is also a good option for lactating and postpartum women.

The Cu T 380A IUD (Paragard), approved for 8 years of use, significantly increases the amount of blood loss with menses (the client already has menorrhagia), whereas the progesterone-releasing Progestasert IUD significantly reduces the amount of blood loss. However, the Progestasert IUD needs to be removed every year, and thus it is used only in special cases, such as copper allergy.

Cost of the IUD is less than or equivalent per year and easier to use than other contraceptives. Initial expense is the insertion cost in the office, approximately $450 (less in a public family-planning clinic).

25. (C) The Cu T 380A increases the amount of blood loss in each menstrual cycle. Normal menstrual cycle blood loss is ~35 mL. With a copper IUD, ~60 mL is lost per cycle. If the client develops heavy menses, check the Hgb and Hct (you may also consider ordering a serum ferritin,

which is a more sensitive marker for iron deficiency anemia). If any of these indicators are low, start an iron supplement (ferrous gluconate is less constipating than ferrous sulfate). Menstrual cycle pain (dysmenorrhea) may be greater (which this client has). The Progestasert IUD reduces amount of blood loss with menses ~25 mL per cycle. Progesterone-releasing IUDs also decrease menstrual cycle pain (dysmenorrhea).

PID is a serious, potentially life-threatening problem and is not considered a nuisance side effect. It can occur during the first few weeks following insertion. With this client a barrier method may be preferable as it reduces PID risk. PID risk is great in women who have more than one sexual partner and whose partners have other sexual partners. IUDs do not protect against STDs. It is unknown whether IUDs increase the risk of acquiring HIV. The effect of the IUD on the endometrium may create a host environment favorable to HIV transmission. Further study also needs to be done to determine if the greater amount of menstrual bleeding with the IUD facilitates HIV transmission.

26. (A) The female condom can be inserted just before intercourse or up to 8 hours before. The female condom should not be used with a male condom too. The female condom can be used with oil-based lubricants because it is made out of polyurethane, not latex. However, oil-based lubricants may cause vaginal infections.

27. (C) The cervical cap has the advantage of being able to be in situ ahead of time and provides effective birth control protection for 48 hours. There is no need to add spermicidal cream or gel regardless of the number of times of coitus (unlike the diaphragm). The female condom can be inserted immediately before intercourse or up to 8 hours ahead. The diaphragm may be inserted immediately before intercourse or up to 6 hours ahead.

28. (C) The efficacy of the female condom as a barrier method is an important factor not only in the role of family planning but also as a physical barrier for the prevention of STDs and HIV. Price ($2.00 each) may limit the acceptance of the female condom.

29. **(C)** Contraceptive protection of vaginal contraceptive tablets and suppositories begins 10–15 minutes after insertion and remains effective for no more than 1 hour. Contraceptive protection with foam, jellies, and creams is immediate and remains effective for at least 1 hour.

30. **(B)** Spermicides reduce STD risk and have been associated with a decrease in cervical cancer.

31. **(B)** Nonoxynol-9 is the active ingredient in most spermicides. It interferes with the sperm membrane. Octoxynol is another spermicidal agent available.

32. **(A)** With typical use of spermicides 21% of women experience an accidental pregnancy within the first year of use. With perfect use 3% experience pregnancy within the first year. Typical use for condoms is 12% in the typical user and 5% in perfect user.

33. **(A)** Failing to use another applicator with each act of intercourse is a common error. Other common errors are using too little foam, failing to shake the foam can vigorously enough, and failing to recognize that the foam bottle is empty.

34. **(A)** Latex condoms are the most effective barrier contraceptive for preventing STDs and HIV. Both synthetic condoms and skin condoms prevent pregnancy by blocking the passage of sperm. Lambskin condoms are not recommended for STD protection as the surface is porous and viruses have been shown to pass through, including hepatitis B, herpes simplex virus, and HIV. Latex condoms should not be used with oil-based lubricants such as baby oil, cocoa butter, Vaseline, or mineral oil.

35. **(C)** Condoms are typically used sporadically and/or incorrectly. The single most important message is to use the condom every time. The condom provides extra protection to cervical cap and diaphragm users.

36. **(A)** Immediately insert spermicidal foam or gel into the vagina. Postcoital contraception may be used. Condoms should not be filled with liquid or air. Every condom is pretested before distribution.

37. **(B)** The flat-spring diaphragm would be contraindicated in a patient with a cystocele as the gentle spring strength is indicated for women with very firm vaginal muscle tone. The arching spring rim has a very sturdy rim with firm spring strength and can be used in patients with cystocele, rectocele, or lax vaginal muscle tone.

38. **(C)** FDA-approved patient labeling recommends a followup visit and Pap smear after the first 3 months of use. Routine visits can then occur on an annual basis but size checks should occur after a weight gain or loss of 10 lb, after an abortion, and following childbirth and cessation of breast-feeding.

39. **(A)** Checking for cervical cap dislodgment is the correct way to assess for cervical cap efficacy. If dislodgment does occur, the patient should leave the cap in its found position, add an applicator of spermicidal gel or cream into the vagina, and consider using postcoital contraception. The cap should be reassessed for proper fit.

40. **(C)** Changes in menstrual pattern are the most common reasons women discontinue Norplant in the first year of use. Approximately 70% of women experience a change in bleeding pattern. The most common changes are an increased number of days of amenorrhea, light intermittent spotting, or heavy bleeding. The patient should be counseled in these changes in advance of the Norplant placement. Three therapeutic approaches are available in management of this side effect: using low-dose combined oral contraceptives, nonsteroidal antiinflammatory drugs, and exogenous estrogens such as Estrace or Premarin. The clinician must discuss the impact of irregular, unexpected bleeding on specific life events such as sexual practices, exercise patterns, and other activities as part of preinsertion counseling.

Women using Norplant complain more frequently of weight gain than loss, but findings are variable and confounded by changes in diet, exercise, and aging. An increase in appetite can be attributed to the androgenic activity of levonorgestrel and the patient should be counseled about appetite changes. This is not a common reason to discontinue Norplant. Research findings do show an association between hormonal contraception and depression and mood changes. Although other variables such as situational stress are confounding, meticulous history taking that includes personal and family history of depression must be considered prior to Norplant insertion. When significant depression does occur following Norplant insertion, removal may be considered. This is not the major reason women discontinue Norplant in the first year of use.

41. **(B)** Ovrette is the progestin-only pill containing norgestrel. A suitability test is attempted where side effects that could potentially lead to Norplant removal might be predicted if a woman uses a progestin only pill for 2 or more cycles prior to Norplant insertion. Possible indications for a trial of Ovrette include concern for the following: acne, weight gain, depression, and allergy to levonorgestrel. Changes in menstrual pattern are not predicted using a suitability test.

42. **(A)** Idiopathic intracranial hypertension has been associated with oral contraceptives, Norplant, and pregnancy. Papilledema may be bilateral or unilateral and is the cardinal symptom of increased intracranial pressure. Other symptoms include severe, unremitting headaches, transient visual obscurations, pulsatile tinnitus, nausea, vomiting, and dizziness. This condition seems to be more common in women who weigh 20% more than ideal body weight.

43. **(A)** The pregnancy rate in women discontinuing Depo-Provera injections is considered within normal limits. The delay to conception is about 9 months after the last injection. Circulating levels of levonorgestrel (Norplant) become unmeasurable 48 hours following removal. The pregnancy rates of post-Norplant users are comparable to those of women not using contracep-

tion or attempting to get pregnant. If the patient wanted to make immediate plans for pregnancy following discontinuation of a method, the best choice would be Norplant, where the average rate of pregnancy approximates the normal population, ie, success by 6 months.

44. **(C)** The most important goal of Norplant insertion is proper placement of the six capsules in the subdermal space and parallel to the surface of the upper arm in a fan-shaped pattern with the proximal tips close together at the insertion site. The importance of proper placement is to aid in easy removal when necessary. The patient's perception of pain is her greatest concern during the Norplant insertion. Using xylocaine 1% buffered with sodium bicarbonate can decrease the local burning associated with xylocaine use. Complete pre-Norplant education as well as viewing the Norplant video can help to decrease the patient's fears.

45. **(B)** Levonorgestrel levels are undetectable 48 hours following removal of the capsules and normal ovulatory cycling can resume immediately resulting in immediate risk of pregnancy.

46. **(A)** Since Natasha is a 36-year-old smoker, the optimal choice for bleeding management would be nonsteroidal antiinflammatory drugs. Oral contraceptives are another treatment choice for management, which is very effective as long as the hormones are taken. The patient must be counseled about use, side effects, and risks of oral contraceptives. The bleeding may return following cessation of oral contraceptives. This method would be contraindicated in Natasha's case as she is a smoker over age 35 years. Although Premarin therapy is another acceptable option, one would consider alternative methods prior to choosing estrogen therapy with its known embolic events.

47. **(C)** The risk of pregnancy is highest during the 3 days prior to ovulation. During this time the rates for pregnancy range from 15 to 26%. The risk of pregnancy with one act of intercourse ranges from 0 to 26% depending on where in the cycle the exposure occurs in relation to ovulation. Coitus 5 days before: likelihood, 0;

4 days before, 11%; 3 days before, 20%; 2 days before, 15%; 1 day before, 26%; day of ovulation, 15%; 1 day after ovulation, 9%; 2 days after ovulation, 5%; 3 days after ovulation, 0 (Hatcher et al, 1994).

48. **(B)** The most common postcoital emergency contraceptive pill method is the "Yuzpe" regimen, two medication treatment doses, taken 12 hours part, totaling 200 µg of ethinyl estradiol and 2.0 mg norgestrel, or 1.0 mg levonorgestrel. Ovral, 2 tabs taken 12 hours apart, is frequently used. Other brand name combination OCs, which require 4 doses taken 12 hours apart, are Lo/Ovral, Nordette, or Levlen; and Triphasil or Tri-Levlen (yellow pills only).

49. **(B)** Emergency postcoital contraceptive pill treatment is highly effective and fails to prevent pregnancy in 0.5% of cases.

50. **(A)** The first dose should be given as soon as possible. There is no need to wait until the next morning, thus the term "morning-after" pill can be misleading. Treatment is most effective if given within 12–24 hours after unprotected coitus. Treatment is not likely to work if delayed longer than 72 hours.

51. **(A)** RU 486 blocks the normal action of progesterone, thereby interfering with implantation of the fertilized egg. RU 486 can also induce menses if implantation has already occurred. The drug has been shown to be 96% effective within the first 9 weeks following LMP when combined with a prostaglandin.

52. **(A)** The term *lower urinary tract infection* includes cystitis (infection of the bladder) and urethritis (infection of the urethra). The symptoms of acute lower UTI (cystitis) are dysuria, urgency, and frequency with or without low back discomfort. Upper tract infection (pyelonephritis) is suggested by flank pain and associated systemic symptoms, which may include nausea, vomiting, or fever and chills. Differentiation can be difficult and up to one third of women with symptoms suggestive of simple cystitis may have unrecognized involvement of the upper urinary tract.

53. **(A)** Studies have indicated that spermicide can increase the risk of bacteriuria with *E. coli*, possibly due to an alteration in normal vaginal flora.

54. **(A)** *Neisseria gonorrhoeae* usually has an abrupt onset and needs to be ruled out in the client with a new sexual partner. The differential diagnosis includes urethritis caused by *N. gonorrhoeae* (acute onset of symptoms) or chlamydia (gradual onset of symptoms). Urethritis is the most likely diagnosis when pyuria is present without bacteriuria in a woman presenting with dysuria.

Dysuria does not necessarily imply a UTI. In taking the history it is important to determine if the symptoms start inside the body with the onset of voiding (urethrocystitis) or occur after the urine washes over the vulva or perineum (vaginitis), and if there are associated vaginal sores ("splash effect") such as in herpes, acute monilial vulvovaginitis, trichomoniasis vulvitis, trauma, or chemical irritants (chemical vulvitis). A sexual history is important in women presenting with dysuria as increased sexual activity is associated with lower UTI ("honeymoon cystitis").

55. **(B)** A cost-effective approach is to confirm the presence of bacteria and pyuria. A urine culture is not necessary in the nonpregnant women who presents with typical symptoms and findings on urinalysis. A follow-up urine culture is not needed unless symptoms persist or recur after treatment.

56. **(A)** Pyuria and bacteriuria with or without hematuria are diagnostic findings on urinalysis. The leukocyte esterase dipstick can detect significant pyuria in up to 95% of cases.

57. **(A)** In simple cystitis the majority of UTIs are caused by facultative anaerobic organisms that colonize the lower gastrointestinal (GI) tract. *Escherichia coli* (*E. coli*) is the most common organism and accounts for 85% of all uncomplicated, community-acquired UTIs. Other gram-negative organisms such as *Klebsiella* or *Proteus* are seen less frequently. Gram-positive organisms such as *Staphylococcus saprophyticus* account for 10% of infections.

In contrast to the simple cystitis, in complicated UTIs there is a higher incidence of infection with other gram-negative organisms such as *Pseudomonas, Serratia, Proteus,* or *Klebsiella.* Gram-positive organisms such as *Staphylococcus* and enterococci are seen (especially after instrumentation of the urinary tract).

Factors that suggest the presence of a complicated UTI are pregnancy, indwelling bladder catheter, recent urinary tract instrumentation, functional or anatomic abnormality of the urinary tract, diabetes, immunosuppression, recent antimicrobial use, hospital-acquired infection, and symptoms for longer than 7 days' duration.

58. **(B)** A 3-day regimen is preferred and has a cure rate comparable to 7-day treatment but without the added cost and potential side effects (rashes, monilial vaginitis, diarrhea).

59. **(C)** In an annually screened population, an ASCUS Pap smear may be repeated in 4 months. The National Cancer Task Force advises that a woman with an ASCUS Pap smear have repeat Pap smears at 4-month intervals for 24 months. If the patient has another ASCUS Pap smear within that period, colposcopy is advised. Acetic acid washing of the genitalia is not a highly sensitive screen for evidence of HPV, which is associated with precursor lesions and cervical cancer. Acetowhitening of the genital tract may also be associated with monilial vaginitis or recent intercourse. Colposcopy referral would be the optimal choice. Since the patient has not had a Pap smear for 4 years, she has lost most of the benefit of the actual screening process. The clinician would also be concerned about her prior history of dysplasia for which evaluation and follow-up are unclear. An ASCUS Pap smear may be related to several etiologic causes, ranging from inflammation and repair to cancer. The main dilemma with the ASCUS Pap smear is that a definitive cause of the cytologic abnormalities cannot be determined and furthur followup is necessary.

60. **(C)** Prior history of a precursor lesion is the major risk associated with cervical cancer. Most

critical is the knowledge that the etiologic agent is a sexually transmitted disease and the incidence of precursor disease is widely prevalent in the young, sexually active population. Teen women have the highest prevalence rates of precursor lesions. Rates of precursor lesions decrease in women as they increase in age. Smoking women have twice the relative risk when compared to nonsmoking controls in association with risk of cervical cancer. The role of oral contraceptive use in association with cervical cancer has not been proven, although recent research has noted an increased frequency of adenocarcinomas in young women who take oral contraceptives.

61. **(C)** Comprehensive counseling and education about genital self-exam are the appropriate steps in management. The incubation period of HPV disease is estimated at 3 weeks to 8 months. Clinical expression of most lesions will occur within that time frame. However, the etiology and course of HPV is not clearly understood. Reevaluation in 6 months should include reexamination of the genital tract, Pap smear, and sexually transmitted disease risk assessment and appropriate testing. Speculoscopy is an adjunctive screening of the transformation zone of the cervix. The clinical goal is to identify areas of abnormal whiteness on the cervix following application of acetic acid and use of an optic magnifying lens and chemiluminescent illumination. The manufacturers claim it increases the sensitivity of the Pap screen when used as an adjunctive tool. At the present time this is not considered a standard screening process. The role of screening for viral subtypes in the absence of abnormal cytology or clinical evidence of a lesion is unclear. The added information of a positive result does not predict the clinical progression of the virus or lesion development. New technology and protocols are being developed that will address use of viral testing and typing in the clinical setting.

62. **(C)** Allergic vulvitis is not associated with vulvodynia. Freidrich defined vulvar vestibulitis syndrome as "severe pain on vestibular touch or vaginal entry; tenderness to pressure localized within the vulvar vestibule and

physical findings confined to vulvar erythema of varying degrees." The cause is poorly understood but considered multifactorial.

63. **(B)** Chronic and acute pain involving or limited to the vulvar vestibule is one of the main features of this syndrome. Physical examination involves using a saline moistened Q-tip and lightly palpating the vulvar tissue to assess areas of involvement. The clinician then diagrams the areas of tenderness. This evaluation is performed at every visit to assess for clinical improvement or change. Touch or pressure seems to exacerbate the symptoms. History may include asymptomatic intervals and only pain when the vulvar tissue is touched as with sexual stimulation, penetration, tampon or pad use, bicycle riding, or clinical examination.

64. **(C)** Meticulous history taking is the first step in the evaluation of vulvodynia. Particular attention should be paid to the identification of a sentinel event that coincided with the symptoms. Review of all prior medical records, symptom profile, treatments and self-care interventions, support systems, sexual activity, impact on lifestyle, and current status should be included. History of incest and sexual abuse should also be explored, although sexual abuse is not consistently associated with this syndrome. History of back injury or back surgery should also be noted as this can be associated with pudendal neuralgia. Colposcopic evaluation should be considered as one of the steps in the evaluation of this syndrome. Biopsies should be performed to identify dermatoses such as lichen sclerosus, lichen planus, or vulvar intraepithelial neoplasia. Evidence of vulvar ectasia may also be confirmed by colposcopic exam. Vaginal flora must be evaluated initially and during all subsequent visits. This is done by noting the characteristics of the secretions and by microscopic examination to rule out infections and assess for balance of the flora. A pH test and whiff test should be performed routinely.

65. **(B)** Intersitial cystitis is associated with vulvodynia. Intersitial cystitis is a disorder characterized by burning pain of the bladder and urethra that may be exacerbated by high-oxalate foods, vulvar pain, and stress. Evaluation includes a cystoscopic exam. The bladder wall will appear hemorrhagic in the absence of bacteria or urinary tract pathogens. Treatments vary and do not consistently resolve the chronic symptoms.

66. **(C)** Vulvodynia is a burning pain which appears to begin suddenly as a result of a trivial insult to the tissue (ie, yeast infection, antibiotic use, childbirth). Once the pain loop is established, the symptoms persist long after the initiating insult is removed or resolved. This pain loop seems to be sympathetically maintained. Histology studies are usually normal but may reveal nonspecific chronic inflammation. Skin changes include atrophy of the vulvar tissue or presence of nonspecific erythema or ectasia. Dysesthesia refers to the alterations in nerve fiber sensitivity such as reflected by hyperalgesic foci, which hurt sharply with even soft pressure. This sympathetically induced pain seems to respond well to drugs that influence the conduction of neurologic impulses within the central nervous system. Tricyclics, calcium channel blockers, and clonidine can help to suppress sympathetically maintained pain syndromes. Fluconazole is considered a treatment of choice when the patient has a history of prolonged or cyclical candidiasis or has taken numerous topical antifungals in association with initial onset or exacerbation of the symptom complex. Another theory is associated with developing a candida hypersensitivity when numerous antifungals have been taken and no evidence of yeast appears on clinical exam or through testing but symptoms of vulvar burning, pruritis, and inflammation exist.

67. **(B)** Amitriptyline may be included as a treatment option to decrease the sympathetically maintained pain loop that is associated with vulvodynia and seems to respond well to tricyclic antidepressants. The patient must be alerted to the sedating effects of the drug prior to use. Surgical excision of vestibular tissue may decrease the symptom complex in 50% of the cases but is not considered a first choice in treatment. Neuromuscular rehabilitation using a biofeedback program looks like a promising

alternative in pain management and resolution of symptoms for these patients.

68. **(B)** The Pap smear is the most appropriate screen as the majority of cervical cancers and precursor states are associated with the human papilloma virus. At least 80 subtypes of the virus have been identified and have been divided into low (eg, HPV 6 and 11) and high (HPV 16 and 18) subtypes. Low- and high-risk lesions can affect the external genitalia and cervical, vaginal, urethral, and anal tissue.

69. **(C)** Laryngeal papillomatosis is a rare consequence of vertical transmission of HPV subtypes 6 and 11, which is characterized by multiple warts on the larynx of children. Juvenile laryngeal papillomatosis (JLP) can cause significant morbidity and can be fatal. Aggressive treatment of external genital warts before delivery is assumed to decrease risk of transmission. Cesarean section has not been demonstrated to prevent JLP and is not routinely indicated.

70. **(B)** Genital HPV infection resulting in external lesions is most often transmitted by sexual contact. The risk of being infected with a genital HPV subtype and developing lesions after sexual contact is unknown. Primary disease is estimated to develop 4–6 weeks after exposure, though interval and frequency of recurrence is unknown. Exposure to the virus may not result in lesion development. Variability of lesion development, transmissibility, and unpredictable recurrence rates make identifying the primary source of infection challenging.

71. **(C)** Lichen sclerosus is the most common of the vulvar dystrophies. The term *dystrophy* is defined as a general heading that includes all disorders of the vulvar epithelium that lead to white surface changes. The dystrophies may be subdivided into three groups depending on clinical and histologic characteristics: lichen sclerosus, hyperplastic, and mixed lesions. Atypia is sometimes noted in the latter two groups. Topical corticosteroids are the main therapy for the hyperplastic dystrophies. If the patient is diagnosed with lichen sclerosis, topical 2% testosterone in a petrolatum base is the preferred treatment. Progesterone cream is an alternative if the side effects of testosterone are intolerable. This is also the treatment choice for children with lichen sclerosis.

In the past, histologic examination of radical vulvectomy specimens found adjacent white lesions with disordered epithelial structure existing with carcinoma. This led to the assumption that white changes preceded cancer. At the present time there is no evidence to conclude that a causal or associative relationship exists. Occasionally white lesions and cancer do coexist. Prospective studies show that the likelihood of carcinoma developing within a preexisting area of benign white change is less than 5%.

72. **(B)** Lichen sclerosis is characterized by vulvar tissue appearing thin and shiny with a crinkled appearance. Initial adhesions may be observed between the labia minora and majora and surrounding tissue. The pattern is usually symmetrical and may produce butterfly or figure eight configurations. If regular intercourse or penetration fails to occur, the introitus may shrink and contract. The cause of this dystrophy is unknown. Patches of similar skin change may be observed on the trunk, neck, and extremities. The most common group affected is postmenopausal women, although lichen sclerosis is found in women in the reproductive age group and in men and children as well.

73. **(A)** Pruritus is the cardinal presenting symptom, with the goal of therapy being to reduce the pruritus and subsequent scratching. Topical corticosteroids are the treatment. The fluorinated compounds are applied twice daily and will cause lesion regression in approximately 4–8 weeks. Eurax can be added to the steroid to decrease pruritus. Once the lesion is resolved completely, recurrence is rare if the irritant has been identified and removed from the patient's environment. Common irritants include laundry products and synthetic underwear fabric. Burning is not commonly associated with hyperplastic dystrophies but may occur secondary to trauma and excoriation subsequent to continuous scratching. Thickening and whitening of the vulvar tissue may be noted by

the patient during genital self-examination but is not considered the primary symptom.

74. **(A)** Mixed dystrophies have a slightly higher rate of atypia when compared to the hyperplastic lesions. The reason for this is unknown. Biopsies for histologic interpretation are a necessary step in evaluation of this patient. The patient must be followed up long term and biopsies taken of any recurrent lesions. The mixed dystrophy may be treated in the following way. Topical corticosteroids are applied to the entire vulva for 6 weeks to resolve the hyperplastic areas, followed by testosterone therapy to reverse the lichen sclerosis. Another option that is equally effective but may take longer for lesion resolution is to use corticosteroid and testosterone preparations on alternative days. This treatment may take up to 2 years but one can often avoid the side effects associated with use of testosterone cream. If atypia is present, the more rapid treatment is preferred.

75. **(C)** Clinically Paget's disease appears as a velvety, red lesion with sharp borders and white islands of hyperkeratosis. It may also appear as bright pink with a scaly eczematoid surface. This syndrome must always be considered in the differential diagnosis of a woman over 60 years old, and biopsies should be taken in cases of persistent vulvitis and/or lesions. Paget's disease is largely confined to the Caucasian population with the median age at diagnosis of 65 years. The major significance of this disease is its role in associative malignancies. If Paget's disease of the vulva is diagnosed, all other sites of potential malignancy must be evaluated and ruled out. These sites include the breast, apocrine sweat glands, cervix, and gastrointestinal tract.

76. **(C)** The primary management of this disease is surgical incision of the entire vulva to the level of the subcutaneous fat. Multiple sections of the entire specimen are submitted to rule out adenocarcinomas of the sweat glands. Shallow skinning procedures run the risk of missing small foci of adenocarcinoma. Routine follow-up is critical due to the high rate of recurrence. Regular visits should occur at 6-month intervals for at least 2 years. Recurrent

soreness or pruritus should alert the clinician to possible recurrence. Steroid therapy may mask the symptoms as well or lead to false assumptions of improvement by the patient and clinician. Biopsies must be routinely performed on any persistent vulvar lesion. It is speculated that patients with Paget's disease delay seeking medical help for up to 2 years. Any patient presenting with a subjective history of a vulvar lesion persisting longer than 3 months must be considered for biopsy prior to treatment.

77. **(C)** The following three symptoms must be present to diagnose PID:
   1. Abdominal direct tenderness
   2. Tenderness with motion of the cervix and uterus
   3. Adnexal tenderness

78. **(C)** To confirm the diagnosis of PID, one of the following must also be included:
   1. Gram stain of cervical or vaginal discharge showing gram-negative intracellular diplococci
   2. Temperature > 38°C
   3. Leukocytosis > 10,000
   4. Purulent material from peritoneal cavity by culdocentesis or laporoscopy
   5. Pelvic abscess, induration, or mass on bimanual exam or ultrasound

79. **(C)** Aggressive management of pelvic inflammatory disease is often recommended to reduce the risk of sequelae. A patient may be managed on an outpatient basis if she meets the criteria for PID but does not have evidence of peritonitis. She should be reevaluated and examined in 48 hours. If no clinical improvement is noted, intravenous antibiotic therapy must be considered. Hospitalization is advised in the following cases:
   1. Signs of peritonitis or a surgical abdomen
   2. Pregnancy
   3. Dehydration
   4. Adolescent
   5. Pelvic abscess
   6. HIV
   7. High fever, elevated white count, or signs of sepsis
   8. Noncompliance with outpatient regimen

80. **(C)** Pelvic inflammatory disease commonly occurs following a menstrual period and is characterized by fever, nausea, and abdominal pain. The clinical manifestations include marked tenderness of the cervix, uterus, and adnexa. The adnexa may be enlarged and a pelvic mass present. Disseminated gonorrhea can lead to an arthritis–dermatitis syndrome characterized by polyarthralgia, tenosynovitis of elbows, wrists, or knees, purulent monoarthritis, and skin lesions. This develops 1 or more weeks following initial exposure.

81. **(B)** The two major sequelae associated with PID are ectopic pregnancy and infertility. Other complications include adhesions, tubo-ovarian abscess formation, and chronic pelvic pain. A single, mild episode of PID will cause infertility in approximately 13% of women. Two episodes leave 35–50% of women infertile, and a third episode increases the incidence to 75%. PID increases the risk of ectopic pregnancy 6–10-fold.

82. **(B)** Chlamydial infection is the most common sexually transmitted disease. It is responsible for 10–40% of acute PID and 25% of urethral syndromes. Chlamydia also causes conjunctivitis and pneumonia in newborns infected with the organism. Chlamydia lacks a typical presentation in upper tract infection, and often the symptoms of abdominal and pelvic pain are mild. Typical symptoms can include abdominal and pelvic pain, dysuria, postcoital bleeding, dyspareunia, and vaginal discharge. On examination the woman may have a normal abdominal exam and mild pelvic tenderness or a surgical abdomen with peritoneal signs. Speculum exam may reveal the cervix to be inflamed, eroded, or friable to touch. Cervical discharge may or may not be present.

83. **(C)** Chlamydial PID has been associated with Fitz-Hugh–Curtis syndrome, an infectious perihepatitis characterized by right upper quadrant abdominal pain. An abdominal examination must always be included when one suspects sexually transmitted disease and/or PID.

84. **(A)** Trichomonas discharge may appear bubbly on speculum exam and there may be punctate petechiae in the genital tract or a "strawberry" cervix (seen with the naked eye in 30% of cases and with a colposcope in all cases). Trichomonads can be seen on the saline wet prep with many wbc's. An anaerobic protozoan, trichomonads can also be seen on routine Pap smears.

Trichomoniasis is transmitted principally through sexual exposure (onset with or following menses) though it is not a reportable venereal disease in the United States. Male partners need to be treated also. Trichomonas is commonly seen in women with peak incidence at 15–40 years. Length of incubation is 7 days on average. Complications include bartholinitis, urethritis, and cystitis.

85. **(A)** Metronidazole (Flagyl), 2 g orally in a single dose. Alternative regimen is metronidazole 500 mg 2 × per day for 7 days.

86. **(A)** Clue cells (epithelial cells with bacteria attached so the cell border cannot be visualized) are seen in bacterial vaginosis (BV). BV is a mixed aerobic and anaerobic infection where the total bacteria in the vagina increase 100–1000-fold, but with no real inflammatory response (thus no leukocytes on wet prep). Background flora consist of small rods and cocci with reduced or absent lactobacilli.

In both BV and trichomoniasis the pH is elevated so this is not a helpful diagnostic clue.

87. **(A)** BV has a positive whiff test or amine odor when the discharge is mixed KOH. A positive whiff test is highly indicative of BV. Other diagnostic criteria for BV are pH > 4.5, clue cells on microscopic exam, and homogeneous discharge. BV was formerly called nonspecific vaginitis and Gardnerella vaginitis. Gardnerella is found in up to 60% of normal vaginal cultures. Thus, vaginal cultures are considered unreliable.

88. **(C)** There is no consensus regarding treating the asymptomatic woman except in cases of women planning to have invasive procedures such as endometrial biopsy, hysteroscopy, IUD insertion, or hysterectomy due to an increased risk or upper genital tract infection. Male partners are generally not treated.

Symptomatic women should be treated. BV has numerous associated diseases. Gynecologic problems include UTIs, postoperative infection, cervical dysplasia, nonpuerperal endometritis, and PID, because the microorganisms that cause upper genital tract infection are also those that colonize the vagina and cervix. Obstetric-associated diseases include chorioamnionitis, premature labor, premature rupture of membranes (PROM), and postpartum endometritis. Pharmacologic treatment options include oral antibiotics and local vaginal Rx.

89. **(C)** The percentage of CD4 lymphocytes is the best predictor of disease progression and prognosis. Individuals with CD4 cell counts greater than 500 are usually asymptomatic and have a low risk of developing an opportunistic infection. Exceptions are tuberculosis, cervical abnormalities, recurrent bacterial pneumonias, or superficial Kaposi's sarcoma. Patients with CD4 counts below 100 have a high risk of developing an AIDS indicator disease. Antiretroviral therapy is not routinely initiated until CD4 counts drop below 500. Prophylactic therapy is not recommended when the CD4 counts are above 500. These counts should be repeated every 3–4 months.

The pulmonary system is most frequently involved in HIV-related opportunistic infections. The diagnosis of AIDS is often made on the basis of a PCP infection. Prophylactic therapy is now recommended for all patients with CD4 counts of less than 200/mm^3.

90. **(C)** Live, attenuated vaccines such as polio, typhoid, yellow fever, and vaccinia should not be given. The exception is live measles vaccine, which can be given according to the recommendations for HIV-negative persons. Preventive care for HIV patients should include administration of pneumococcal vaccine as a one-time dose. Pneumococcal pneumonia is the leading bacterial pneumonia in HIV-infected patients. The vaccine has been shown to stimulate antibody levels high enough to provide protection, especially in individuals with early symptomatic disease. Hepatitis B vaccine should also be given in hepatitis B surface antigen and antibody-negative patients because of the increased risk of developing chronic hepatitis.

91. **(C)** HIV-positive women do show a higher prevalence of cervical intraepithelial neoplasia than do their noninfected counterparts. The role of routine colposcopy screening in the absence of abnormal cytology in regularly screened patients is still controversial. Invasive cervical cancer is relatively uncommon in HIV-positive women. HIV-positive women are at increased risk for noninvasive vulvar intraepithelial neoplasia even in the absence of cervical disease. Regular vulvar inspection is an important part of the screening process. Colposcopic evaluation and biopsies should be performed on atypical lesions. The protocol for Pap screening is Pap smears every 6 months for the first year and then annually in the absence of HPV history or active infection.

92. **(A)** *Pneumocystis carinii* pneumonia (PCP) is the most common opportunistic infection in AIDS patients. Prophylaxis with the preferred agent Bactrim (trimethoprim-sulfamethoxazole) prevents infection and prolongs life. In the HIV patient, PCP prophylaxis continues for life.

HIV patients are at risk for toxoplasma gondii encephalitis if they have been previously exposed to the organism. This is not as common as PCP. A serology for IgG antibodies to *T. gondii* indicates that the patient is at risk for reactivation later in the course of HIV disease. CDC guidelines include toxoplasmosis prophylaxis for all HIV-infected persons with CD4 counts below 100. Trimethoprim-sulfamethoxazole is the treatment of choice. Although not as common as PCP, tuberculosis infection can occur at any CD4 count and can worsen the prognosis of the HIV-infected patient. All HIV-positive patients should have a Mantoux skin test unless they have had a previous positive skin test or earlier treatment for tuberculosis. A positive TB test should be worked up for evidence of disease.

93. **(B)** Petra's partner should be encouraged to return for testing 12 weeks from the date of at-risk behavior. If the test is negative, he should have a repeat test in 3 months. Counsel him in HIV prevention strategies and give an explanation of the limitations and interpretations of HIV testing. Antibodies to HIV usually

appear 6–12 weeks after infection but may take as long as 6 months to appear. The diagnosis of HIV infection is based on detection of anti-HIV antibodies by the enzyme-linked immunosorbent assay (ELISA), confirmed by the Western blot method. Her partner may elect to have an immediate test but must understand the limitations of testing and that a negative test at this time may not reflect a recent infection with the HIV virus. If the partner has participated in high-risk behavior in previous relationships, he should be encouraged to have immediate testing.

94. **(B)** The most likely diagnosis is HSV. HSV is the most common cause of vulvar ulcers. Type 1 is usually associated with oral nasal infections ("cold sores"), and HSV type 2 usually causes infections of the vulva, vagina, cervix, and anus. But either type can be found in either location. In general, type I usually occurs above the waist and type II below the waist though HSV-1 is found in 10–30% of pelvic infections. This client was infected from the herpetic lesion on her partner's lip during oral relations. Her presentation is classic for a primary herpetic infection. Ulceration of or near the urethra causes dysuria.

HPV are painless lesions, as is a syphilitic chancre. It would be important to screen this client for other STDs. Finding one venereal disease suggests the probability that the patient has a second STD of the lower genital tract. Her history is not consistent with a syphilitic chancre.

95. **(A)** After exposure, the incubation period is 48 hours to 7 days before the onset of a primary herpes infection. The infected sexual partner may or may not have active lesions, and may be entirely without symptoms, yet shed viral particles.

96. **(B)** Culture is the most sensitive method to detect herpes infection. Herpes cultures have about an 80% sensitivity. It is best to get the specimen from the vesicle rather than crusted lesions, late in the course. Pap smear can be used to detect giant cells associated with herpes infection, but there is a 30% false-negative rate. Serologic tests for herpes show only that the patient has been exposed in the past.

97. **(B)** Antiviral medication will reduce the duration of viral shedding, the time to healing, the duration of symptoms, and the clinical course of the disease. After initial infection with genital herpes, herpes recurs at unpredictable times, as the virus is latent and resides in the dorsal root ganglion of S2, S3, and S4 and within the autonomic nerves along the uterosacral ligaments. Recurrences are more common in times of stress or immunosuppression—for example, in pregnancy, in patients on chemotherapy, or in leukemic patients.

Treatment of recurrent infections needs to be started within 2 days of the onset of lesions and may shorten the clinical course 1–2 days. Patients who experience recurrences 6 times or more per year may receive continuous-treatment prophylaxis (provided liver function tests are normal). Safety in pregnancy has not been established. There is no cure for herpes.

98. **(B)** Diabetes is a risk factor for vaginal yeast/fungal infections due to an increase in vaginal glucose levels. Women with recurrent vaginal yeast infections should have a glucose screen with a random blood sugar (BS; HIV screen if HIV risk factors are present). If the BS is elevated, follow up with an FBS. Other risk factors for candida which interfere with the normal lactobacilli ("good germs") are systemic glucocorticoids, antibiotic use, pregnancy, immunsuppressive disorders (including AIDS), and possibly OCs. Estrogen appears to encourage the growth of *Candida* species, though low-dose OCs may be less likely to be a co-factor than high-dose OCs. The majority of women with an occasional vaginal yeast infection do not have any of these risk factors.

Candida are normal flora of the skin, mouth, intestinal tract, and vagina but cause disease when there is an abnormal overgrowth. *Candida* are not considered to be transmitted sexually in most cases, but male partners can acquire the organism and be a source of reinfection.

99. **(A)** If pruritus is absent, then candidiasis is unlikely. Candidiasis can have minimal vaginal discharge. Less than half of patients present with adherent white thick curd-like patches of the vulva and vaginal walls (thrush patches). Vaginal pH is 4.5 or less.

Dysuria (burning with urination) is common and is usually due to burning of the vulva during urination (vulvar dysuria). Dyspareunia on insertion may be present due to vulvar erythema. Women usually do not complain of an offensive odor but may describe a "yeasty" odor. Rash is not the most common symptom but a red florid vulvar rash and erythema (resembling "diaper rash" may be present in severe cases).

100. **(B)** KOH wet prep is 80% sensitive. KOH destroys the cellular elements, sparing the *Candida albicans* species. *Candida albicans* are dimorphic fungi that grow as oval budding yeast cells and chains of cells or filaments (hyphae). It is difficult to visualize *Candida* species on the saline smear.

In a symptomatic patient take a culture with Nickerson's medium or Sabouraud dextrose if the KOH is negative. Since *Candida* colonize the vagina without causing symptoms, treatment is not recommended if the culture is positive but the client has no symptoms.

The Pap test is not considered sensitive as a diagnostic test.

101. **(A)** Candida albicans is present in the majority of vaginal yeast infections.

102. **(A)** Normal pH is relatively acidic. Lactobacilli (Lbs) are the predominant organisms in the normal vaginal flora. Lbs produce lactic acid, which results in normal acidic pH. pH is increased during menses, after exposure to alkaline semen, and by hormonal changes.

This patient is midcycle and an increased amount of vaginal discharge is normal in ovulatory cycles (stretch "spinbarkeit" mucoid, slippery discharge).

All of the STDs thrive in an alkaline pH so it can serve as a good screening tool in the office. However in estrogen deficiency the pH is usually greater than 6.

103. **(C)** Routine tests are pH, wet prep, and amine ("whiff") test. The addition of 10% KOH does not change the odor (the amine test) in normal physiologic leukorrhea. Wet prep of normal discharge has superficial epithelial cells, lactobacilli (string-like bacteria), and occasional leukocytes.

Note that the microbiology of the flora are complex, made up of mixed aerobic and anaerobic organisms. Organisms considered to be pathogenic in the vagina (such as *Escherichia coli*, *Bacterioides fragilis*, *Staphylococcus aureus*, group B streptococci, and *Candida* species) in some circumstances are considered to be normal.

Since the patient is a virgin, gonorrhea and chlamydia screen would not be indicated.

104. **(B)** The primary lesion of lymphogranuloma venereum (LGV) is a painless, 2–3 mm vesicle or vesicopapule at the site of inoculation, which may not be detected by the patient. The secondary stage is characterized by an inguinal syndrome of acute lymphadenitis with buboes (enlarged matted nodes) occurring 1–4 weeks following the primary lesion. A sensation of inguinal pain or stiffness followed by swelling in the inguinal region is the most common clinical presentation. Adenopathy may subside spontaneously or lead to abscess formation and rupture.

105. **(A)** LGV is caused by *Chlamydia trachomatis*.

106. **(C)** The LGV complement fixation test level of 1:64 is considered diagnostic. The definitive test requires isolating *Chlamydia trachomatis* from the lesion or inguinal bubo aspirate. This is not done routinely. Suspected cases should be promptly treated with doxycycline 100 mg po bid for 21 days. Prompt examination of the sexual partner is also required.

107. **(C)** The molluscum contagiosum lesions have a typical appearance and can be diagnosed by inspection in the majority of cases. If there is any question about diagnosis, the central cheese-like core can be expressed onto a glass slide and examined microscopically. Large inclusion bodies that occupy most of the cell cytoplasm are characteristic. This is not done routinely. If the lesion is inflamed, it may resemble folliculitis or herpes and will complicate diagnosis by inspection.

108. **(B)** The standard treatment for molluscum contagiosum consists of scraping open the papule with a sterile needle or scalpel, express-

ing and removing the contents, and cauterizing the base. The patient is instructed to take sitz baths, keep the area clean and dry, and follow up in 1 month to identify new lesions.

109. **(C)** Sexual contact is not necessary for transmission as the above disease can be spread by fomites or autoinoculation. Lesions of the face, trunk, and extremities are more commonly seen in children. The lesions of adults are generally located on the genitals and thighs.

110. **(A)** Syphilitic chancre is painless. A nonpainful and minimally tender ulcer that is not accompanied by inguinal adenopathy is likely to be syphilis. Chancroid is very painful, as are herpes lesions. Syphilis is the second most common cause of genital ulcer disease. The ulcer has smooth margins and a firm and palpable (indurated) border. The ulcer base is clean with a serous, not purulent, exudate.

111. **(A)** The causative agent of syphilis is *Treponema pallidum. Hemophilus ducreyi* is the causative organism of chancroid or soft chancre. *Neisseria* (gram-negative intracellular diplococci) are the causative agent in gonorrhea.

112. **(B)** Secondary syphilis usually occurs about 4–10 weeks after the chancre appears.

113. **(C)** Generalized maculopapular rash affecting the trunk and limbs, including the palms of the hands and the soles of the feet, is a feature of secondary syphilis. Condylomata lata are fleshy lesions with a pearly gray appearance that may occur on the genitalia. Buboes occur with lymphogranuloma venereum (LGV) rather than syphilis.

114. **(A)** Benzathine penicillin, 2.4 million units IM. Quinolones are not active against *Treponema pallidum.* Metronidazole is used in the treatment of trichomonas and bacterial vaginosis.

115. **(C)** Patients with a first-degree female relative (mother or sister) with endometriosis have 7 times increased risk of developing the disease. Endometriosis does not discriminate on the basis of age, socioeconomic status, childbearing history, or ethnicity. However, it is more likely to occur and progress in women with early menarche, menstrual flow exceeding 7 days, and cycles less than 27 days. Risk factors for developing endometriosis are also any condition that obstructs the outflow of menstrual fluid—such as scar tissue on the cervix as a result of treatment for cervical cancer.

116. **(C)** A definitive diagnosis can be made only by visualization of the implants in the pelvis, usually by laparoscopy. The role of laparoscopy is to confirm the diagnosis and extent of the disease and to treat visible disease with surgery, laser, or electrocautery. The ovary is the most common site and is affected in approximately 40% of cases; thus the menorrhagia. The next most common site is involvement of the cul-de-sac and uterosacral ligaments—a fixed retroversion—and is associated with deep dyspareunia. Women suspected of having the disease should be referred to a gynecologist for definitive diagnosis and continued treatment.

Even though endometriosis is associated with the classic triad of symptoms and infertility, there is a wide spectrum of presentations not necessarily correlated with the extent of disease but possibly correlated with the site. One third of women are asymptomatic and are diagnosed with endometriosis during an infertility workup. But dysmenorrhea or acute and chronic pelvic pain are the more common presentation. If the genitourinary tract or rectum is involved, patients may experience painful defecation or hematuria (during menses when growths are largest or are bleeding).

CA-125 levels are frequently elevated, but the CA-125 level is neither specific nor sensitive enough to aid in diagnosis.

Neither history nor the physical exam are pathognomonic for endometriosis. An exam performed near the time of menses may reveal only mild tenderness. Tender uterosacral ligaments or tender nodules in the posterior cul-de-sac are suggestive of the disease. In advanced cases the uterus may be retroverted and fixed and the posterior vaginal fornix narrowed.

117. **(B)** The goal of pharmacologic intervention is relief of pain and resorption of endometrial implants, return to fertility, and pregnancy if desired. This client has no childbearing plans.

118. (B)

REVIEW OF GONADOTROPIN-RELEASING HORMONE AGONISTS (GNRH-A)

Gonadotropin-releasing hormone agonists suppress pituitary gonadotropin secretion.

- **Leuprolide acetate (Lupron)** 0.5–1.0 mg sc qd ×6 months or 3.75–7.5 mg IM q 28–60 days. Amenorrhea occurs at 4–6 weeks, Rx for 6 months; recent data show 3 months may be adequate.

- **Nafarelin acetate (Synarel)** nasal spray can be used instead. 1 spray (200 µg/spray) into one nostril q AM and the other nostril q PM × 6 months
  - *Side effects:* Related to the hypoestrogenic state such as hot flushes, insomnia, vaginal dryness, mood swings, depression, weight gain, decreased breast size, decreased libido, and fatigue (all of which are reversible). GnRH-a may interfere with calcium and bone metabolism (may be only partially reversible).
  - *Contraindications:* Known or suspected pregnancy, undiagnosed vaginal bleeding, hypersensitivity to GnRH, breast-feeding
  - *Note:* Expensive; provide supplement of calcium carbonate 1000–1500 mg. Barrier contraception is recommended during Rx and for the first cycle after Rx.
  - Recent data on "add-back" therapy shows that adding norethindrone and conjugated estrogens may decrease the side effects.

Other Rx
- **Danazol** 100–800 mg qd. Danazol is an androgen derivative. Danazol has been used most widely either alone or in combination with surgical intervention to suppress symptoms. An 800 mg dose is given as two 200-mg tablets bid × 6–9 days beginning in day 5 of menses. It is expensive and requires long-term administration. Barrier contraception is recommended during Rx with danazol and with the first menstrual cycle after Rx.
  - *Side effects* reflect the hypoestrogenic state and the androgenic and anabolic effects. Hot flushes, vaginal dryness, emotional liability, weight gain, fluid retention, and acne are more common side effects. There is a lower incidence of hirsutism, decreased breast size, and voice changes.
  - *Contraindications:* Liver disease, hypertension, CHF, renal impairment, or pregnancy
- **Progestogens:** As effective as danazol.
  - Dose: **Medroxyprogesterone acetate (Depo-Provera)** 100 mg IM q 2 weeks ×4 doses, followed by 200 mg IM for 4 additional months and 30 mg po qd ×6 months
  - *Side effects:* Breakthrough bleeding (BTB), depression, delayed fertility, headache, dizziness, weight gain
  - *Contraindications:* Known or suspected pregnancy, undiagnosed vaginal bleeding, desiring return to fertility immediately after finishing Rx
  - Note: Provide supplement of calcium carbonate 1000–1500 mg qd.
- **Combined OCs:** Suppress cyclical hormonal response of endometrial implants and eventual resorption of the tissue.
  - Dose: 1 tab qd continuously for 6–12 months with BTB. Can give conjugated estrogen 2.5 mg qd ×1 week. Can also increase OC dose to 2 tabs qd if BTB.

119. (B) Adenomyosis is also known as "internal endometriosis" as the endometrial glands and stroma within the endometrium extend diffusely into the myometrium. During the menstrual cycle, this lining grows and develops in response to hormones, but at the time of the menstrual period it cannot shed and bleeds within itself in the myometrium. Menorrhagia is the most common symptom; the enlarged uterus can cause pelvic discomfort, bladder and bowel discomfort, deep dyspareunia, and in some cases a noticeable abdominal mass. It is rare for the uterus to be larger than 12–14 weeks size.

Of multiparous women in their 30s and 40s, 10–20% develop this condition, but it does not occur postmenopausally.

Treatment is based on the patient's age, severity of condition, and desire to maintain fertility. There is no specific treatment to resolve adenomyosis. Use of GnRH agonist therapy, NSAIDs, or OCs can be helpful.

Referral to a gynecologist for hysterectomy may be indicated for intractable, symptomatic adenomyosis including severe dysmenorrhea or uterine enlargement greater than 10 weeks.

120. **(A)** Uterine leiomyomas are benign neoplasms that arise from the uterine smooth muscle and are the most common (one out of every five women and as many as one out of three African American women) pathologic conditions of the female genital tract. They are rarely malignant.

Risk is less with increased parity and with greater age at last term birth. Smoking decreases risk (due to decreasing estrogen levels) and obesity increases risk (due to increasing estrogen levels). OC use is not associated with an increased risk of myomas.

121. **(C)** Fibroids are classified according to their location in the uterus.

- Submucous—protruding into the uterine cavity
- Intramural—within the myometrial wall
- Subserous—growing toward the serous surface of the uterus
- Interligamentous—located in the cervix or in between the folds of the broad ligament

122. **(A)** The most common presenting complaint is menometrorrhagia. The patient may or may not be anemic and may or may not have dyspareunia. Usually clients are asymptomatic; however, symptoms present as the tumor grows in size. Common symptoms are pelvic pressure, bloating, pelvic congestion, a feeling of "heaviness," urinary frequency, dysmenorrhea, dyspareunia, constipation, and less commonly pain (pregnant women complain more of pain).

If the fibroid outgrows its blood supply, degeneration results and acute pelvic pain occurs.

123. **(A)** For women with abnormal bleeding that is thought to be secondary to fibroids, endometrial evaluation is necessary to rule out the presence of endometrial hyperplasia or cancer. Pap smear should be obtained as part of the routine

workup. CBC would be ordered depending on the severity of the hypermenorrhea.

Patient's bleeding can be managed by Depo-Provera q 3 months and is a useful conservative Rx for submucosal fibroids once premalignant or malignant conditions have been ruled out.

Rx of choice GnRH agonists (sc, IM, or intranasal). With Rx mean uterine size decreases 30–64% after 3–6 months. Relief of menorrhagia, anemia, pelvic pressure, and urinary frequency is obtained after 3 months. When discontinued, myoma and uterine size return to pretreatment size in 3–4 months.

124. **(A)** Vaginal ultrasound can differentiate uterine leiomyomas from ovarian neoplasm in most cases. However, MRI is considered superior to ultrasound as it can be difficult to distinguish between submucous myomas and endometrial polyps.

Occasionally a hysterosaplingogram is used to evaluate the site and location of a submucous fibroid prior to hysteroscopic resection.

125. **(B)** Leiomyomas develop during the reproductive, hormonally active years and regress after menopause.

126. **(B)** After age 35 there is a tendency for serum estradiol to decrease, most probably reflecting a reduction in the responsive cohort of follicles at the beginning of the cycle. This results in less feedback inhibition, which raises the FSH levels and leads to a shortened follicular phase. In the late 40s the luteal phase may also become inadequate with lower progesterone levels and early dissolution of the corpus luteum resulting in further shortening of the cycle. Anovulatory cycles and missed cycles are the events that occur later in the perimenopausal cycle following a decrease in estrogen and progesterone levels and further shortening of the menstrual interval.

127. **(A)** Atrophic epithelial changes at the onset of menopause reverse rapidly as evidenced by a clinical and symptomatic improvement in 6–8 weeks. Protracted estrogen deprivation results in a permanently contracted genital tract due

to irreversible loss of the deeper supporting connective tissue, vasculature, and musculature in the dermis. When the underlying dermis is involved, the changes require longer term therapy. One may see tissue responsiveness and improvement in 12–24 months. Atrophic tissue changes that have connective tissue involvement may not respond to therapy. The role of the clinician is to identify atrophic changes as menopause begins and to formulate a plan with the patient that may involve estrogen therapy or alternative treatments. Severity of symptoms is not always predictable and nonestrogen options must be addressed in order that the patient be enabled to make an informed choice.

128. **(A)** Hot flashes occur at irregular intervals from occasional to many times per day and may awaken the patient at night. Research has shown that these episodes are objectively identified by altered skin and core temperatures and are closely related temporally to episodic secretion of gonadotropins by the pituitary gland. Hot flashes precede an increase in FSH and LH by just a few minutes. It is theorized that the FSH and LH spikes are increased in amplitude, not frequency, starting in perimenopause and this exaggerated excitation may spread to adjacent thermoregulatory centers in the hypothalamus, hence setting off the hot flash.

129. **(B)** The vaginal pH becomes more alkaline as glycogen production decreases. Mucosal atrophy and the alteration of acidity in the vagina may result in symptoms of itching, discharge, and localized burning or tenderness. Many women complain of decreased lubrication with intercourse and dyspareunia.

130. **(A)** Postmenopausal osteoporosis is a common disorder characterized by an increase in bone resorption relative to bone formation, generally in conjunction with an increased rate of bone turnover. The decrease in bone mass leads to an increase in the susceptibility to fractures, which results in substantial morbidity and mortality. Known risk factors include a positive family history of osteoporosis. The incidence of fractures is greater in

Caucasian than in African-American women, probably reflecting greater peak bone mass at maturity in blacks. Clinically significant fractures are five to eight times more common in women than in men. Cigarette smoking, sedentary lifestyle, prolonged bedrest, alcohol abuse, nulliparity, diabetes mellitus, and chronic glucocorticoid therapy are all factors that increase the risk of osteoporosis.

131. **(C)** The measurements of spine and hip are most predictive of osteoporosis risk and often correlate. Hip fractures significantly increase the risk of morbidity and mortality. DEXA measurements may not be as accurate for vertebral assessment when compared to the quantitative computed tomography scanning. QCAT is more precise but requires relatively high levels of radiation exposure. Wrists can be used as a measurement of osteoporosis risk but are not considered as accurate as measurements of the spine and hip.

132. **(C)** When contemplating estrogen therapy at menopause for the prevention of osteoporosis, bone density less than 2.5 standard deviations below the mean for normal women has been recommended as the marker for initiation of therapy. Values 1 SD above the mean indicate that the risk of developing osteoporosis is quite low. Age-corrected average measurement reflects an assumed average loss depending on the age of the woman and not her optimal level of bone mass.

133. **(B)** Women should be encouraged to participate in a program of moderate progressive, weight-bearing exercise to activate osteoblastic bone formation. Women have an increased need for calcium and vitamin D supplementation during menopause. The recommendation is 1500 mg of elemental calcium per day and 400 IU of vitamin D. Other suggested steps include reduction of caffeine and alcohol intake and smoking cessation. Decreasing dietary protein intake will also help to promote a positive calcium balance.

134. **(B)** Premarin 0.625 mg po daily is the minimum dosage of conjugated estrogens com-

bined with calcium supplementation and a weight-bearing exercise program to provide good protection against postmenopausal osteoporosis. Data from the Postmenopausal Estrogen–Progesterone Interventions trial suggest that combined homone therapy protects as well as unopposed estrogens. Estradiol 2 mg po daily is an adequate dose. ERT should begin as soon as possible after natural menopause or oophorectomy because estrogen slows the rate of bone loss but cannot restore bone mass to pretreatment levels.

135. **(A)** During the first 5 years following menopause calcium loss is primarily through vertebral (trabecular) bone. After 5 years following menopause, calcium loss occurs equally from the hip, long bones, and spine. Eventually fractures occur. Crush fractures initially predominate, causing back pain, height loss, and a stooped posture. It has been estimated that if a Caucasian woman lives to be 90 years of age, she has a 32% chance of sustaining a hip fracture.

136. **(B)** When LDL levels were studied it was found that LDL levels increase with age in both sexes but between ages 45 and 55 (menopause). LDL cholesterol in women increases significantly and exceeds the level in men after age 50. It appears that the LDL levels rise when estrogen is deficient. Therefore, it appears that the cardioprotective effect of endogenous estrogens is in part mediated by its influence on LDL. Cross-sectional measurements in men and women of various ages have shown that mean levels of HDL cholesterol are higher in women than in men at every age and either do not decrease or decrease slightly after menopause. HDL levels appear to be independent of endogenous estrogen levels and menopause.

137. **(B)** It is now believed that estrogen has the ability to inhibit the deposition of LDL cholesterol in the wall of the artery. The PEPI trial also found that decreased fibrinogen levels were found among women in all treatment groups compared to placebo ($p < 0.001$), although no significant differences were found among the treatment groups. Estrogen is also thought to improve vasomotor tone and blood flow.

138. **(A)** Serum FSH and LH levels should be mesured to see if this patient is menopausal. The levels should be drawn on day 7 from the LMP. An FSH level above 30–40 mIU/mL indicates menopause. The standard procedure at the current time for evaluation of irregular bleeding is the endometrial biopsy (EMB). This office procedure provides the clinician with a pathology sample that can rule out endometrial hyperplasia and cancer. This would be an appropriate diagnostic intervention for this patient, who presents with 6 months of irregular bleeding. Transvaginal ultrasonography of the endometrium can measure endometrial depth. Endometrial thickness of less than 3 mm reflects low estrogen levels and has not been associated with hyperplasia. The normal postmenopausal endometrium is a thin, linear echogenic structure that is usually less than 5 mm thick. A depth of less than 5 mm indicates a very low risk of cancer. A thick endometrium of 5–8 mm thickness warrants endometrial sampling and should raise the suspicion of hyperplasia. This is not considered the standard diagnostic test but could be used in association with the EMB to assess endometrial thickness.

139. **(B)** The Nurses Health Study did indicate a modest elevation of risk for current users as compared to women who had never used estrogen (R.R. = 1.3: 95% CI, 1.1–1.5). The greatest risks noted in the aforementioned study were noted in women using hormones for 5–9 years (R.R. = 1.5; 95 % CI, 1.2–1.70) and longer than 10 years (R.R. = 1.5; 95% CI, 1.2–1.8). Cardiovascular benefits are well documented, consistent, and substantial. A women who takes ERT has a 50% less chance of death from coronary heart disease than a woman not taking estrogen. Coronary heart disease is the most significant disease in this country and has significant mortality and morbidity outcomes. As the leading cause of death, it exceeds the number of deaths associated with breast cancer. It is to the benefit of the patient that we provide accurate information

and individual risk assessments so that optimal choices can be made on an individual basis.

140. **(A)** Hereditary ovarian cancer syndromes affect 1% of women in the United States. These syndromes are inherited in an autosomal dominant pattern. Three hereditary ovarian cancer syndromes are identified: site-specific ovarian cancer, the most common familial syndrome restricted to families with history of ovarian cancer only; breast and ovarian syndrome, where breast and ovarian cancer exists in extended family pedigrees; and the Lynch II syndrome, which includes early-onset nonpolyposis colon cancer, endometrial cancer, upper gastrointestinal cancer, renal, pelvic, and ureteral cancer, and ovarian cancer. Women in these families may have a lifetime risk of developing ovarian cancer that is as high as 50%. This compares to a 5–7% risk if a woman has one or two family members with ovarian cancer.

141. **(B)** The clinician should order an ultrasound to identify and measure the adnexal mass. The two largest ovarian cancer screening studies using transvaginal ultrasound showed specificity of 98% and 97%. Transvaginal ultrasound has better quality and resolution than the transabdominal ultrasound and eliminates the need for a full bladder.

142. **(A)** The CA-125 is a cell surface antigen that is used to monitor women with known epithelial ovarian cancer. Elevated CA-125 levels prior to surgery that rise during followup are a reliable predictor of relapse. A low stable CA-125 level does not exclude relapse. CA-125 has been found to be elevated in other conditions, including breast, colon, ovarian, and cervical cancer. Nonmalignant conditions associated with elevated levels include endometriosis, fibroids, PID, pregnancy, cirrhosis, pericarditis, and menses.

143. **(C)** The greatest risk factor for endometrial cancer (EC) is unopposed estrogen use, which increases the risk of EC fivefold. The risk accelerates with higher doses of estrogen replacement therapy and persists for up to 5 years following discontinuation of use. Unopposed estrogen is associated with endometrial hyper-

plasia, which is the precursor of endometrial cancer. The histologic diagnosis of endometrial adenomatous hyperplasia increases the risk of developing cancer by 25%. The presence of atypia in association with adenomatous hyperplasia increases the risk by 50%. Adding concurrent use of progesterone decreases the risk to nearly that of women not taking HRT.

144. **(C)** Risk factors for endometrial cancer include polycystic ovarian disease, early menarche, late menopause, nulliparity, and infertility. Other factors that may be associated with chronic high levels of estrogen are increasing age, obesity, and menopause. Diabetes and hypertension are also risk factors. Women with other cancers have a slight increased risk of endometrial cancer. Oral contraceptives offer a protective effect. The relative risk of women on oral contraceptives is 0.4 when compared to women with no history of OC use.

145. **(B)** Dilatation and curettage is the definitive diagnostic procedure for endometrial cancer. It provides the clinician with a histologic sample but it may miss other noncancerous causes of bleeding such as fibroid tumors or polyps. Currently, an alternative choice would be in office endometrial sampling using a disposable plastic pipette along with a transvaginal ultrasound with measurement of the endometrial lining thickness. Women with negative endometrial samplings and an endometrial lining thickness of less than 5 mm seem to have a very low risk of endometrial cancer.

146. **(B)** The International Federation of Gynecology and Obstetrics (FIGO) has defined a surgical staging system for endometrial cancer. Stage 1B is defined as disease limited to the endometrium including invasion of less than half of the myometrium. Cervical involvement, depth of invasion of the endometrium, spread beyond the uterus, and poor histologic differentiation are poor prognostic signs.

147. **(A)** The treatment of stage 1A is total abdominal hysterectomy and bilateral salpingoophorectomy. Women with endometrial cancer require close followup. Two thirds of recurrences

occur within 3 years. Women who have stage 1 cancer plus poor risk factors may be offered adjunctive radiation therapy.

148. **(B)** The clinician should gather menstrual information with the goal of attempting to quantify menorrhagia. The most clinically significant information is gained by inquiring about changes in bleeding pattern as compared to normal cyclical intervals, bleeding amount, duration, and associated symptoms such as pelvic cramping. Menstrual pad counts are used as an approximate measurement of blood loss, but this method correlates poorly with actual recordings of loss in scientific studies.

149. **(C)** Dysfunctional uterine bleeding (DUB) is a diagnosis of exclusion and is not associated with systemic disease, pregnancy, pelvic inflammation, genital tumors, or other anatomic lesions. Disruption of the cyclic release of GnRH, FSH, or LH can result in chronic anovulation and abnormal bleeding patterns. Dysfunctional uterine bleeding with anovulation in the perimenopausal woman is associated with decreased sensitivity of the ovary to gonadotropin stimulation. The most common presentation of DUB is breakthrough bleeding. FSH stimulates the ovary to produce estrogen. Inadequate amounts of estrogen are produced, resulting in the suppression of an adequate FSH/LH surge. The follicle continues to make estrogen without progesterone and the endometrium is fragile and readily breaks down, resulting in irregular bleeding.

150. **(B)** Women who present with abnormal bleeding after the age of 35 years should have endometrial sampling to rule out endometrial carcinoma, hyperplasia, or other uterine lesions, such as a submucous myoma or endometrial polyp. The endometrial biopsy is the gold standard procedure. Prospective studies of endometrial biopsy results show reliable differentiation between benign disease and endometrial carcinoma. The procedure can be done on an outpatient basis and is generally well tolerated using a nonsteroidal antiinflammatory drug as premedication.

151. **(A)** A mass in an adolescent is almost pathognomonic for a fibroadenoma, especially in African-Americans. If breast symptoms are unilateral or there is a palpable mass, refer the patient for further evaluation. Women with fibrocystic changes usually present with bilateral nodularity and increased tenderness or pain prior to menses. The nodularity may be generalized or localized and tends to be more pronounced in the upper outer region.

Fat necrosis is a rare lesion that can occur at any age, with half of patients with a previous history of trauma to the breast. On physical exam there is usually a hard, tender, mobile, indurated mass with irregular borders that may be accompanied by skin or nipple retraction. It may be seen after segmental resection and radiation therapy.

152. **(C)**

DESCRIPTION OF TANNER'S STAGES OF BREAST DEVELOPMENT

STAGE	DESCRIPTION
Stage 1	Preadolescent
Stage 2	Breast bud; elevation of nipple, enlargement of areola
Stage 3	Increased subcutaneous breast tissue, smooth contour of breast and areola
Stage 4	Secondary mound of areola and nipple above breast contour
Stage 5	Mature, recession of areola to form a breast with a smooth contour

153. **(A)** Ultrasound can be of value to determine if the mass is solid as in a fibroadenoma or cystic. Mammograms are usually not obtained in young girls this age as the tissue is so dense it is difficult for the radiologist to interpret. Thermography is generally not used in primary care and needs to be refined further before it can be considered reliable.

154. **(C)** Fine-needle aspiration cytology in the office can provide the definitive diagnosis. Excision under local anesthesia is usually recommended for a fibroadenoma.

155. **(A)** Fibrocystic breast changes, also termed fibrocystic breast disease (FBD), are so common

that they are also called *physiologic nodularity*. FBD usually presents as diffuse nodularity, but can also present as a discrete mass. The patient may have cyclic pain and tenderness. Data unequivocally show that OC users are less likely to develop benign breast tumors (such as fibrocystic changes and fibroadenoma) with the low-dose formulations than women not using the pill. Pills do not have a protective effect against breast lesions diagnosed as atypia on biopsy (which are considered to be premalignant). Nonpuerperal mastitis is a rare condition that usually occurs in late adolescence or middle years. There is a palpable mass—usually an obscure organism. The clinician should rule out syphilis or tuberculosis.

156. **(B)** Hormonal cyclic activity is a physiologic condition. In FBD, bilateral nodularity and increased tenderness or pain may be increased prior to menses. The nodularity may be generalized or localized and found more in the upper outer region. FBD is most common in women 30–50 years old and rare in postmenopausal women (not taking hormone therapy). There are no well-designed studies to support that patients may also experience an improvement of FBD symptoms with reduced caffeine, methylxanthine intake, and sodium intake and use of vitamin E 600 IU/day. However, these are benign treatments and there may be a "placebo" effect. Medications for fibrocystic breast changes, such as Danocrine (danazol), Parlodel (bromocriptine) and Nolvadex (tamoxifen), may be tried to decrease pain and nodularity.

157. **(C)** Breast cancer incidence increases with age. Most women who develop breast cancer do not have an identifiable risk factor other than age. A woman at age 70 has 10 times the risk of developing breast cancer as a woman at 40 years of age. Over 90% of women with breast cancer have no family history.

BREAST CANCER RISK FACTOR REVIEW

- **Reproductive experience:** Risk of breast cancer increases with the age of first full-term pregnancy. To be protective, pregnancy must occur before age 30.
- **Ovarian activity:** Small decrease in risk with late menarche and a moderate increase in risk with late natural menopause (suggests ovarian activity is an important feature). Women who have had an oophorectomy have a lower risk of breast cancer; lowered risk is greater the younger a women is when she has her ovaries removed.
- **Obesity:** Greater risk for breast cancer. Obese women have earlier menarche and later menopause, as well as higher estrogen production rates and free estradiol levels (lower sex hormone binding globulin).
- **Benign breast disease:** FBD is a risk factor *only* if breast biopsy showed evidence of atypical hyperplasia. Risk increased 3–5 times if on biopsy there is atypical hyperplasia.
- **Familial tendency:** Female relatives of women with breast cancer have 2–3 times the rate of general population.

Affected mother or sister	2.3 relative risk
Affected aunt or grandmother	1.5 relative risk
Affected mother and sister	14.0 relative risk

In some families breast and ovarian cancers are inherited; however, only 5–10% of all breast and ovarian cancer can be attributed to the inheritance of a gene associated with high risk. The breast and ovarian cancer gene (BRCA1) associated with familial cancer is on the long arm of chromosome 17, but other genetic alterations have also been observed in breast tumors.

- **Diet:** Fat in the diet—little support.
- **Alcohol:** Almost all studies conclude that moderate drinking increases the risk 40–60%.
- **OCs:** Long-term use not associated with a significant increase in risk of breast cancer after age 45. There is a possibility that a subgroup of young women who use OCs early for more than 4 years has a slightly increased risk (a relative risk of 1.5) of breast cancer that occurs before age 45. The use of OCs does not further increase the risk of breast cancer in women with positive family histories of breast cancer or in women with proven benign breast diseases.
- **DES:** Significant but modest (less than twofold) increase in the risk of breast cancer.

158. **(A)** For all women over 35 with a palpable breast mass *order a diagnostic mammogram.* Mammography either alone or in combination with a thorough clinical breast exam reduces breast cancer deaths, especially in older women.

Diagnostic mammography is used to evaluate women with a breast mass(es) or other breast symptoms (nipple discharge, skin changes), an abnormal or questionable screening mammogram, a history of breast cancer, or breast augmentation. It may also include other modalities of breast imaging such as ultrasound. The diagnostic mammogram may require additional views of the breast.

Ultrasound (US) is less sensitive than mammography as a screening tool for breast cancer. Ultrasound can rarely reveal malignant lesions smaller than 1 cm in size. It is useful to guide the aspiration of lesions and to distinguish cysts from solid masses. US is useful in evaluating clinically palpable masses not visible on mammogram in younger women. Thermography and light scanning (diaphanography or transillumination) have not been shown to be of value and have a high false-positive rate. CT scans deliver too large an x-ray dose and the slices are too thick to detect early lesions. MRI is not practical because of the expense and long scan times.

Screening mammogram is an x-ray exam to detect unsuspected breast cancer at an early stage in asymptomatic women. It usually consists of two views of each breast.

When ordering a mammogram, specify which one is being ordered, as the diagnostic mammogram usually takes more time and generally requires the presence of the interpreting physician.

159. **(B)** The breast mass is most likely a galactocele. Though it is uncommon, a woman may present with galactorrhea and a breast mass. A galactocele is a milk-filled mass caused by over distention and obstruction of a lactiferous duct. Most galactocele develop after cessation of lactation. Galactorrhea is usually white or clear. If the color is yellow or green, consider breast disease. Hormonal secretions usually come from multiple duct openings, whereas pathologic discharge usually comes from a single duct. Galactocele are not risk factors for breast cancer. Withdrawal of milky discharge with evidence of fat globules is diagnostic for galactocele. Fine-needle aspiration (FNA) is often curative.

Puerperal mastitis occurs spontaneously in 2% of all postpartum lactating mothers (both primiparous and multiparous), usually 2–4 weeks postpartum. The mass is warm to the touch, indurated, usually unilateral; the most common etiology is *Staphylococcus aureus.*

Incidence of intraductal papilloma (benign lesion of the lactiferous duct) peaks at age 40. It is usually associated with serous, serosanguinous, or bloody nipple discharge on affected side. On exam of purulent discharge under the microscope, normal fat globules are absent and leukocytes occlude the field. **Any discharge that is blood tinged requires further evaluation.** Benign causes are intraductal papilloma, fibroadenoma, and ductal ectasia.

160. **(A)** In patients with nipple discharge a prolactin level should be drawn to rule out hyerprolactinemia. Hyperprolactinemia is generally defined as persistent elevated prolactin levels of more than 20 ng/mL. Also order a TSH or thyroid profile to rule out hypothyroidism and a CT scan with visual field assessment to rule out pituitary adenoma or other CNS lesion (if the prolactin level is elevated). Note that hyperprolactinemia is a major cause of anovulation and the associated infertility. Neither an SMA 12 nor a CBC would be useful in the workup.

161. **(A)** Note the National Cancer Institute (NCI) and the American Cancer Society (ACS) recommendations differ for women 40–49 but agree for women over 50.

AMERICAN CANCER SOCIETY RECOMMENDATION FOR BREAST CANCER SCREENING

- Teach BSE at 20
- Clinical breast exam every 3 years age 20–40 and every year after 40
- Mammography every 2 years age 40–49
- Mammography every year starting at age 50

THE NATIONAL CANCER INSTITUTE (NCI) SUMMARY OF EVIDENCE FOR BREAST CANCER WITH MAMMOGRAPHY

- Age 40–49 years: No evidence to make an informed decision regarding efficacy of screening
- Age 50 and over: Routine screening every 1–2 years with mammography and clinical breast exam and/or mammograms

162. **(B)** Primary dysmenorrhea occurs in the absence of pelvic pathology (physical exam is normal) whereas secondary dysmenorrhea occurs as a result of some underlying organic pathology. Menstrual pain of primary dysmenorrhea usually begins 6–12 months after establishing ovulatory cycles and the pain lasts typically 48–72 hours. Up to 50–70% of women of childbearing age experience primary dysmenorrhea.

   Pain is usually suprapubic but may radiate to the thighs, groin, and sacrum and may have associated symptoms of nausea, diarrhea, headache, bloating, or breast tenderness (molimina).

   Secondary dysmenorrhea begins with underlying organic pathology. Suspect if pain begins after age 20. The pain is not strictly limited to menstrual phase; onset occurs after adolescence, and severity may increase over time. Most common causes are endometriosis and PID. Other causes are uterine fibroids (leiomyomata), cervical stenosis, ovarian cyst, adhesions, adenomyosis, endometrial hyperplasia, and endometrial cancer.

163. **(B)** NSAIDs are also known as prostaglandin synthetase inhibitors. Regression of the corpus luteum causes a decrease in the progesterone level. Fragmenting endometrial tissue releases the prostaglandins PGF_2 and PGE_2. Prostaglandins cause contractions. Contractions cause hypoxia and ischemia, and pain results.

   The patient should be given a 6-month trial with necessary change in dose and inhibitor. She should start at the first hint of cramps. Because this client does not need contraception, OCs would not be the first choice of medication.

   Aspirin is also a prostaglandin inhibitor but weaker in therapeutic effect than NSAIDs.

164. **(B)** Interstitial cystitis is a syndrome characterized by bladder pain, irritative voiding symptoms (urgency, frequency, nocturnal dysuria), and sterile urine. The etiology of the disease is poorly understood. Numerous studies have failed to identify a causative bacterial, viral, or fungal infection. The consensus at present is that the syndrome is multifactorial and each case must be approached individually. No current treatment approach leads to complete resolution of symptoms.

165. **(C)** Antibiotic regimens do not successfully treat the symptoms of interstitial cystitis unless the patient is having an acute episode of cystitis. Urine cultures should be sent routinely if this is suspected to confirm the growth of bacteria. These cases should be treated with antibiotics and will be curative for the acute episode of UTI.

166. **(C)** Studies show that the full development of the classical symptom complex occurs over a short period of time. The disease did not seem to progress continuously but reached its final stage rapidly and then stabilized at that level. Late deterioration of symptoms is unusual.

167. **(A)** One of two cystoscopic findings must be present to diagnose interstitial cystitis. These are glomerulations or Hunner's ulcer. The evaluation consists of cystoscopic evaluation with bladder distention. Glomerulations, which are pinpoint petechial hemorrhages, must be diffuse and present in at least three quadrants of the bladder. A classic Hunner's ulcer is a discrete bladder ulceration noted upon distention of the bladder and present in a minority of patients.

168. **(B)** One of the major treatments of interstitial cystitis is the intravesical instillation of dimethyl sulfoxide (DMSO). The pharmacologic actions include antiinflammatory and analgesic effects, membrane penetration, collagen dissolution, muscle relaxation and mast-cell histamine release. The drug is commonly given weekly for 6–8 weeks with approximately 50% of patients reporting relief of symptoms.

169. **(A)** A pelvic examination and pregnancy test are warranted to rule out pregnancy. If the

pregnancy test is positive a pelvic ultrasound may be considered. Ectopic pregnancy must be considered in the differential diagnosis as the patient has a history of pelvic inflammatory disease and irregular bleeding. Pelvic adhesions and irritable bowel syndrome must also be considered as part of the differential diagnosis once pregnancy is ruled out.

170. **(B)** Recurrent vaginitis is not commonly associated with pelvic pain. Recent research has found bacterial vaginosis associated with increasing the risk of endometritis following operative procedures. A microscopic wet mount, pH test, and whiff test of vaginal exudate would rule out this possibility.

171. **(C)** Laparoscopy can diagnose endometriosis, adhesions, fibroids, and pelvic masses. Lysing adhesions is often effective in relieving symptoms of pelvic pain. When laparoscopic examination is normal, other causes of chronic pelvic pain must be investigated.

CAUSES OF CHRONIC PELVIC PAIN

Gastrointestinal: Irritable bowel syndrome
Constipation
Diverticulosis
Urologic: Urethritis/urethral
syndrome
Cystitis
Interstitial cystitis
Chronic or recurrent
pyelonephritis
Gynecologic: Ovarian cysts
Endometriosis
Adhesions
Chronic PID
Uterine or ovarian cancer
Nerve entrapment syndromes
Musculoskeletal pain syndromes

172. **(A)** Vaginismus is an involuntary contraction of the pubococcygeus muscles, introitus, and lower third of the vagina. It exists in a primary and secondary form. In the primary form the muscle spasms exist prior to attempted penetration. In the secondary form penetration

with intercourse or while inserting an object such as a tampon may precede vaginismus. The muscle spasm is totally involuntary. The underlying dynamic associated with vaginismus is fear of vaginal penetration. Sexual abuse has been associated with vaginismus. The clinician should take a sexual history and elicit information about age at coitarche, past sexual experiences, and evidence of abuse. History of incest abuse may not be conciously known by the patient. Repression of the sexual abuse experience (by a family member) is often a mechanism of defense by a survivor. Vaginismus management is often best comanaged by a clinician and a psychotherapist. The psychotherapist can explore past history of sexual abuse and provide guidelines for management. Secondary vaginismus may be the result of dyspareunia that has resulted from recurrent or recalcitrant vaginal infections. The proper evaluation would be to treat the ongoing infection and when it is resolved, counsel the patient in desensitization techniques. This is often long-term therapy.

173. **(B)** Psychotherapy referral to an individual with expertise in sexual dysfunction would be appropriate. Co-management of the patient by the therapist and clinician would be optimal.

Use of vaginal dilators is a behavioral-modification process where the goal is to decrease involuntary muscle contractions by introducing graduated sizes of vaginal dilators into the vagina without sensations of pain and within patient's control. The patient should be instructed by the clinician in dilator use and relaxation exercises and should return at monthly intervals for evaluation of progress. The woman is given a set of four dilators to take home and is encouraged to place the smallest one into the vagina on a daily basis for 15–20 minutes. The patient is encouraged to do this at a time when she is relaxed and can avoid interruptions. This treatment plan can be highly successful.

174. **(C)** Jana would be diagnosed with sexual aversion disorder. This is defined as extreme repulsion and avoidance of genital contact with self or a partner.

Jana does not seem to have inhibited sexual desire as she admits to feelings of arousal and sexual dreams. Inhibition occurs when a woman lacks desire for sexual activity, sexual dreams, and fantasies. Levine has emphasized that the interaction of biologic drive, psychologic motivation, and cognitive aspiration all play a role in the human state of sexuality. Masters and Johnson's research affirmed the hypothesis that individuals demonstrate sexual consistency over the life cycle. They also found that early onset of sexual activity and frequent orgasms were predictive of continued sexual activity longer in life. The clinician should attempt to evaluate the causes of inhibited or low sexual desire and refer the patient and her partner to a therapist if necessary.

Anorgasmia or anorgasmic is defined as the inability to experience orgasm following sufficient stimulation. Since Jana has no history of masturbation or sexual stimulation, she would not be considered anorgasmic.

175. **(B)** Anorgasmia or the inability of a woman to experience orgasm with sufficient sexual stimulation is the correct definition. The diagnosis of female orgasmic disorder should also include what is reasonably expected for her age, sexual experiences, and current activities and any history of chronic illness, stress, and medication use. Anorgasmia is associated with medication, drug use, and medical conditions. Alcohol and cocaine use may have impact on orgasmic response. The orgasmic response is physiologically governed by the autonomic nervous system in both sexes. Conditions that inhibit orgasm are neurologic disorders, drugs that have impact on the autonomic system, and surgical or traumatic interruption of the neural pathways. Diabetic autonomic neuropathy is a common cause of inhibition of orgasm in women. Interpersonal difficulty and distress is often associated with sexual dysfunction and marital discord. The clinician should note that a history of previous orgasmic response is a good prognostic indicator. A block in orgasmic response may be associated with stressful life situations. Counseling for secondary anorgasmia should include the partner if the patient is willing to include him/her. Counseling should

include addressing the dominant issues, which are often related to life stressors or interpersonal conflicts. Women with primary anorgasmia can be referred for counseling and instructed in sexual stimulation techniques with a partner and with masturbation.

176. **(A)** The patient would be instructed by the clinician in the anatomy and phsiology of the genital tract and associated functions including sexual function and response. The patient would be encouraged to view her own genitals using a hand-held mirror while the clinician identifies the anatomic parts and associated functions. The patient would be instructed in touch and stimulation of the genital area. The initial goal is to enhance relaxation and decrease genital tract spasm. The long term goal is to enable the patient to enjoy sexual stimulation and orgasm. Therapy in Jana's case is considered long term. Partner participation would be discouraged. The patient's fear of pain and need for complete control in starting this therapeutic process would exclude any partner participation at the present time.

177. **(A)** Researchers describe four stages of sexual response: excitement, plateau, orgasm, and resolution. Two physiologic characteristics of sexual excitement are common to all mammals including humans. The first is engorgement and dilatation of genital and pelvic blood vessels by means of increased arterial blood supply. This reaction has a secondary effect on penile erection as the cavernous penile bodies become congested with blood and vaginal lubrication as the perivaginal vasculature becomes engorged. The second physiologic response is increased voluntary muscle tension. Individuals who are sexually excited tend to display muscle tension, restlessness, voluntary and involuntary movements, thrusting, grimacing, and clasping.

One significant difference between men and women is the ability to acheive multiple orgasms during a single sexual episode. Women are physiologically capable of moving from plateau to orgasm one to several times during one sexual event. Men have a refractory period that follows ejaculation. During the refractory period it may be difficult to achieve an erection and subsequent orgasm and ejaculation. The length of the refractory period gradually increases as men grow older. The refractory period may be 5–15 minutes in an 18-year-old and 18–24 hours in a 60-year-old.

The plateau phase consists of sustained engorgement, muscle tension, elevated heart and respiratory rates, and elevated blood pressure that may vary in duration from minutes to hours. The orgasmic phase consists of rhythmic contractions of the pelvic voluntary and involuntary musculature in both sexes. Orgasm is the beginning of relief from the sustained physiologic response in the plateau phase. Resolution is the gradual loss of muscle tension and progressive relaxation and is often associated with a sense of drowsiness and contentment. Blood vessels open to drain pelvic and genital engorgement, and gradually the individual returns to a nonexcited state.

178. **(B)** The patient needs to be examined completely with photographs taken of all injuries. Documentation of contusions, bruises, abrasions, lacerations, bite marks, and swelling should be noted. Examination of the external genitalia and a descriptive assessment of the tissue including the hymen is included. Speculum, bimanual, and rectal exam are necessary to look for signs of trauma, seminal fluid, and infection. Specimen collection should be carried out according to medical and legal guidelines. Providers should offer to call the police but only with the consent of the patient.

179. **(B)** Rape Trauma Syndrome is a set of behavioral, somatic, and psychologic responses to rape. This two-phase reaction has an acute phase, which lasts from 48 hours to several months, and a long-term phase that may last several months to years. Approximately 25% of the rape victims experience severe and long-term symptoms. Women with a history of rape are more likely to receive diagnoses of major depression, alcohol and drug abuse, generalized anxiety, obsessive compulsive disorders, and sexual dysfunction. Sexual assault victims perceive themselves as having poorer health than nonvictims do.

180. **(C)** Sexual assault is a violent crime that has been misperceived by society. Although attitudes are slowly changing and legal reforms reflect our understanding of this violent crime, many still believe that victims invite rape by provocative behavior. Failure to resist the rape has been interpreted as indirect sanctioning or consenting by the victim. Rape has been perceived stereotypically as a physically violent assault, and bruises and wounds are expected to prove that a victim resisted the assault. Although rape is violent, between half and two thirds of victims have no evidence of physical trauma. More than half of victims are submissive when placed in the position of deciding whether there is more danger from the rape itself or from the act of resisting and potential physical harm. Although the social climate is changing, many victims choose not to become involved with the legal system because of these misperceptions.

181. **(C)** Polycystic ovarian syndrome (PCO) is defined as a chronic hyperestrogenic and hyperandrogenic condition associated with anovulation. Up to 90% of women who present with hirsutism and have irregular menses have PCO. True virilization is rare but 70% of anovulatory patients complain of cosmetically disturbing hirsutism. Additional signs of virilization to check for are scalp hair loss, voice deepening, muscle mass increase, and clitoromegaly. Hirsutism is central in distribution and follows the midline of the body.

182. **(A)**

POLYCYSTIC OVARIAN SYNDROME (PCO)

The three cardinal symptoms are menstrual disorders, hirsutism, and infertility. Amenorrhea, oligomenorrhea, or dysfunctional uterine bleeding present in 80% of cases. Hirsutism is seen in 70% of cases and infertility is the presenting symptom in 75% of patients with PCO. Anovulation is a key feature of amenorrhea and presents as amenorrhea in 50% of cases with irregular bleeding and 30% of cases with heavy bleeding.

Obesity has been classically regarded as an important feature of PCO but anovulation can result from many causes. The presence of obesity in PCO is variable and has no diagnostic value. However, the greater the body mass—the greater mass index—the higher the testosterone levels and therefore hirsutism is more common in overweight anovulatory women.

Alopecia and acne are also consequences of hyperandrogenism.

183. **(A)** An increase in androgen levels (usually testosterone) is the primary factor in hirsutism. In the evaluation of this client's hirsutism you would obtain a serum testosterone and a dehydroepiandosterone (DHEAS). Women with hirsutism have increased production rate of testosterone and androstenedione.

As part of the evaluation for anovulation you would also obtain prolactin levels and screen thyroid function. Also consider hyperinsulinemia. In many patients a disorder in insulin action precedes the increase in androgens.

184. **(A)** Anovulatory women have a higher LH; increased androgens result in increased estradiol levels, which further decrease FSH levels (or reverse FSH:LH ratio). The increase in LH stimulates the theca interna of the follicle to produce increased amounts of androstenedione (an androgen), which is responsible for the androgenic features of the disease. Since androstenedione is a major precursor of estrogen, PCO is also a hyperestrogenic disorder.

Though the elevated LH value in the presence of low or low-normal FSH may be diagnostic, the diagnosis can be made by clinical presentation alone. About 20–40% of patients do not have elevated LH levels with reversal of LH:FSH ratio. Some clinicians do not routinely measure FSH and LH in anovulatory patients.

185. **(B)** The risk of endometrial cancer is reported to increase threefold. During the reproductive years anovulation has been associated with three to four times increased risk of breast cancer appearing in the postmenopausal years, though this figure is controversial and further research needs to be done. Supplemental calcium would be recommended in the amenorrheic woman even if no estrogen is prescribed.

186. **(B)** The decision to perform an endometrial biopsy should not be influenced by the patient's age. It is the duration of exposure to unopposed estrogen that is critical.

187. **(A)** Amenorrheic and anovulatory women need to be screened with a serum thyroid-stimulating hormone (TSH) as part of the evaluation. Hypothyroidism may be associated with elevated prolactin levels.

Any woman who has a disorder of ovulation including amenorrhea should have at least one serum prolactin test. If the prolactin is greater than 100 ng/mL, then further evaluation of the pituitary is necessary. Order a CT scan or MRI of the sella turcica to rule out a pituitary tumor.

Women with amenorrhea may present with Cushing's disease—a disorder in which a tumor of the pituitary gland causes the adrenal glands to produce an excess of the glucocorticoid hormones.

II

Obstetrics

Obstetric Cases and Questions

Questions 188–190

A 32-year-old woman presents for her first prenatal visit at 9 weeks. She is gravida 6 para 5 with a history of GDM in her second pregnancy. She is currently on Micronase bid. On physical exam today her blood pressure is 142/90, urine is negative for protein but 2+ for sugar, and she has an 8-week AV uterus.

188. What test should be ordered along with her prenatal profile?

(A) Blood sugar
(B) 24-hour urine for creatinine clearance and total protein
(C) Hgb A_{1c}

189. The patient asks you what she should take for medication to control her diabetes. You tell her to

(A) Continue with Micronase bid
(B) Decrease Micronase to qd
(C) Change to insulin

190. Her Hgb A_{1c} result is 14%; this indicates that

(A) Her blood sugars have been within range.
(B) Her FBS is about 100.
(C) Her blood sugars are very out of control.

Questions 191–193

A pregnant woman presents for her first prenatal exam. On her history she informs you that she works as a preschool teacher.

191. Which screening profile would be ordered?

(A) TB, parvovirus antibodies, varicella, hepatitis B
(B) TORCH
(C) Toxoplasmosis, parvovirus, CMV, HSV

192. At 16 weeks' gestation she may have been exposed to Fifth's disease. The correct test to order is

(A) Parvovirus IGG & IGM
(B) Parvovirus antibodies
(C) TORCH

193. Her test results are as follows: parvovirus IGM > 10, IGG <10, which indicates

(A) Recent exposure
(B) Past exposure
(C) No exposure

Questions 194–197

A 35-year-old primigravida woman presents for initial prenatal exam. Her LMP was 7 weeks ago. On physical exam, her uterus is the size of a cantaloupe.

194. The most likely diagnosis is

(A) Multiple gestation
(B) Single intrauterine pregnancy
(C) Ectopic pregnancy

195. Her risk factors for this diagnosis include all of the following EXCEPT

(A) Age
(B) Parity
(C) Race

196. In twin gestation

(A) AFP cannot be done
(B) AFP can be done
(C) Amniocentesis is the only recommended test

197. Which one of the following statements is true for a twin gestation pregnancy?

(A) Prenatal vitamins should have 1 mg of folic acid.
(B) Prenatal vitamins should have 2 mg of folic acid.
(C) Prenatal vitamins should have 400 μg of folic acid.

Questions 198–200

198. Dizygotic twins are

(A) From 2 ova and 2 sperm
(B) From 1 ova and 1 sperm
(C) From 2 ova and 1 sperm

199. Which twin gestation is at risk for twin–twin tranfusion due to vascular anastamosis?

(A) Dichorionic and diamniotic
(B) Monochorionic and diamniotic
(C) Monochorionic and monoamniotic

200. All the following statements are true about twin pregnancies EXCEPT

(A) One abnormal pregnancy–induced hypertension (PIH) parameter may be enough to decide upon hospitalization.
(B) There is a risk for preterm labor (PTL).
(C) Both fetal heart rates should be about the same.

Questions 201–206

The results of a 32-year-old African-American G1 patient's complete prenatal blood count are as follows: RBC = 3.53 mil, Hct = 33%, Hgb = 11 g, MCV = 111, MCHC = 36%.

201. These results are

(A) Normocytic and normochromic

(B) Macrocytic and normochromic
(C) Microcytic and hypochromic

202. The next important test to order is

(A) Folate
(B) Ferritin level
(C) Hemoglobin electrophoresis (Hgb electrophoresis)

203. Test results are as follows: folate = low, ferritin = normal, Hgb electrophoresis = A1(98%), A2 (1%). The diagnosis is

(A) Iron deficiency anemia
(B) Beta thalassemia
(C) Folic acid deficiency

204. If this client was taking Dilantin, the dose of folic acid should be

(A) The normal amount of 1 mg
(B) A higher dose of 2 mg
(C) A lower dose of 400 μg

205. Risk factors for B_{12} deficiency would include all the following EXCEPT

(A) Gastrectomy
(B) Crohn disease
(C) Alcohol abuse

206. If the client was diagnosed with β-thalassemia trait, she will need

(A) Additional iron supplementation
(B) No added iron supplementation
(C) To be evaluated at 28 weeks to determine iron levels

Questions 207–210

A 40-year-old G2 P1 woman presents for a prenatal exam at 8 weeks from LMP.

207. A mild systolic flow murmur is noted on exam. This indicates

(A) Abnormal finding and need for echocardiogram
(B) Within normal finding
(C) Normal finding but need for echocardiogram

208. Her blood bank sample is O negative with Kell antibodies. You know that the antibody indicates

(A) All is within normal limits
(B) The client needs further testing
(C) You should be concerned about fetal well-being

209. The breast exam reveals a 1-cm firm mass in right upper outer quadrant (RUOQ). The next step is

(A) Breast ultrasound
(B) Mammogram
(C) Repeat breast exam on next visit

210. Screening questions to determine this client's risk for toxoplasmosis should include all of the following EXCEPT

(A) Do you have a cat?
(B) Do you eat raw eggs?
(C) Do you garden?

Questions 211–215

At an obstetric visit a pregnant woman admits to occasional use of cocaine in pregnancy. She is not concerned since she says she did it in her last pregnancy and nothing happened to her or the child.

211. The use of cocaine may put her at risk for all the following EXCEPT

(A) Small for gestational age (SGA)
(B) Abruptio placenta
(C) Placenta previa

212. A urine toxicology screen test can be

(A) Done monthly on urine left for dipstix
(B) Done now and in labor
(C) Done monthly only if patient agrees

213. Intrauterine growth retardation (IUGR) can occur with cocaine use in pregnancy and is usually

(A) Asymmetrical
(B) Symmetrical
(C) Combined

214. The patient also smokes a half pack of cigarettes a day and may be interested in Nicorette or a nicotine patch.

(A) Nicotine patch can be used in pregnancy.
(B) Nicorette gum can be used in pregnancy.
(C) Nicotine patch is not recommended during pregnancy.

215. Alchohol consumption in pregnancy should be limited to

(A) No consumption
(B) No more than 2 drinks a week
(C) No more than 4 drinks a week

Questions 216–220

216. An initial urine culture (C&S) grows > 100,000 *E.coli*. The patient is not symptomatic but has sickle cell trait. The next step would be to

(A) Treat her with a 10-day course of amoxicillin
(B) Repeat the urine C&S
(C) Treat with a 3-day regimen of amoxicillin

217. A pregnant woman develops genital condylomata. The treatment of choice would be

(A) Podophyllum
(B) Condylox
(C) Trichloracetic acid (TCA)

218. A pregnant woman with a history of asthma takes Ventolin and Beclovent inhalers. She can

(A) Continue to use Ventolin inhaler as needed
(B) Use Beclovent inhaler
(C) Use both as needed

219. All of the following are used for management of hyperemesis gravida EXCEPT

(A) Phenergan suppositories
(B) Reglan tablets
(C) Scopolamine patch

220. Atypia on a Pap smear at initial exam would cause you to recommend

(A) Repeat smear at 28 weeks
(B) Colposcopy and Pap smear at 28 weeks
(C) Colposcopy and biopsy at 28 weeks

Questions 221–226

A G2 P1 woman was induced at her first pregnancy due to pregnancy-induced hypertension (PIH). Her baseline blood pressure (BP) for this pregnancy is 110/64.

221. At 32 weeks' gestation she complains of swelling of both feet. Her BP is 120/70, urine dipstix negative/negative, and fundal height 32 cm. You would

(A) Reassure her this is within normal range
(B) Order CBC, platelets, chemistry profile with liver function test (LFT)
(C) Order non-stress test (NST)

222. At 34 weeks' gestation her BP is 132/86, urine is trace protein, swelling is present in ankles and fingers, and her weight is up 2 lb in 2 weeks. You would

(A) Reassure her that she is within normal limits
(B) Order CBC, platelets, chemistry profile with LFTs
(C) Order NST

223. At 36 weeks' gestation BP is 138/84, urine is 1+ protein, weight gain of another 2 lb, and her blood work is as follows:

BUN	18	creatinine	0,8
uric acid	6.4	LDH	282
alkaline phosphate	135	Hct	44.7%
platelets	384		

The diagnosis is

(A) PIH (pregnancy-induced hypertension)
(B) Essential hypertension
(C) Acute fatty liver disease

224. For a more comprehensive exam of this client you would

(A) Check her reflexes for hypoactivity
(B) Evaluate her for orthostatic changes in vital signs
(C) Perform ophthalmologic exam for papilledema

225. Manifestations of PIH include all of the following EXCEPT

(A) Headaches and visual changes
(B) Proteinuria and weight gain
(C) Jaundice

226. All of the following statements about PIH are true EXCEPT

(A) It occurs more frequently in primigravidas.
(B) Chronic disease states such as diabetes have an increased risk for PIH.
(C) PIH occurs more commonly in women between the ages of 20 and 30.

Questions 227–233

Selma is a 27-year-old woman who presents with irregular bleeding. She "had her period at the normal time with a regular flow that stopped and then started again." She now has heavier bleeding with severe left-sided pelvic and abdominal cramping accompanied with dizziness. Her urine home pregnancy test was positive.

227. The most likely diagnosis is

(A) Threatened abortion
(B) Ectopic pregnancy
(C) Blighted ovum

228. Risk factors for an ectopic pregnancy include all the following EXCEPT

(A) History of birth control pill use
(B) Appendectomy
(C) DES exposure

229. Her quantitative beta human chorionic gonadotropin (BHCG) was 1432 mIU/mL. What test would be ordered next?

(A) Repeat BHCG in 48 hours
(B) MRI of pelvis
(C) Transvaginal ultrasound

230. Selma elects to try a nonsurgical protocol. What methotrexate (MTX) medication would be ordered?

    (A) MTX 100 mg/m^2 IV
    (B) MTX 50 mg/m^2 IM
    (C) MTX 100 mg/m^2 IM

231. Five days after receiving MTX, a repeat BHCG is 1500 mIU/mL. This finding is considered

    (A) Abnormal; needs immediate intervention
    (B) Within normal limits; repeat BHCG in 48 hours
    (C) Abnormal; repeat BHCG in 48 hours

232. Selma asks if she should continue taking prenatal vitamins. The best response is to

    (A) Continue with prenatal vitamins; they will provide supplementation
    (B) Stop vitamins; they will interact with protocol
    (C) It would be ok to continue a multivitamin

233. The patient's blood bank sample is as follows: O negative, passive anti-D antibodies. This indicates

    (A) Rh sensitivity
    (B) Need for Rhogam
    (C) Patient has received Rhogam

Questions 234–236

234. On an initial prenatal exam green vaginal discharge is noted; pH > 5.0, with large amount of WBC. The most likely diagnosis is

    (A) Group B streptococcus
    (B) Trichomonas
    (C) Bacterial vaginosis (BV)

235. The management of this patient would be to

    (A) Treat patient and partner after 12 weeks with po Flagyl
    (B) Treat patient and partner with E-Mycin
    (C) Treat patient with MetroGel

236. Her RPR result is 1 : 34 with a negative FTA indicating

    (A) Current infection
    (B) Past infection
    (C) False positive

Questions 237–240

237. On initial prenatal exam, the client reports a history of thyroid problems or possible hyperthyroidism. The most sensitive test to check thyroid function is

    (A) sTSH
    (B) FT$_4$
    (C) T$_3$

238. An important test to be ordered on this patient would be

    (A) Serum calcium
    (B) Thyroid stimulating immunoglobulins (TSI)
    (C) Triiodothyronine

239. The plan of care for this client should include

    (A) Biophysical profile (BPP) starting at 30 weeks
    (B) Non-stress testing (NST) starting at 30 weeks
    (C) Ultrasound at 28 weeks

240. On initial prenatal exam, the client is taking Synthroid for an underactive thyroid. An important screening test would be

    (A) TSH
    (B) Total T$_3$ and T$_4$
    (C) Thyroid stimulating immunoglobulins

Questions 241–243

A 28-year-old Haitian client who is 8 weeks pregnant has received bacillus Calmette-Guérin (BCG) in the past.

241. A purified protein derivative (PPD) test

    (A) Should not be done
    (B) Should be considered positive if induration ≥ 5 mm
    (C) Should be considered positive if induration ≥ 10 mm

242. She works as a patient care assistant and questions you about hepatitis B vaccine. Your response would be

    (A) Not advised in pregnancy
    (B) Wait until after the first trimester
    (C) Can begin immunizations

243. An important screening test for this woman would be

    (A) Sickledex
    (B) Hemoglobin electrophoresis (Hgb E)
    (C) CBC with MCV

Questions 244–250

Jamie is a 31-year-old G1 at 15 weeks' gestation who elects to have an alpha-fetoprotein test. You recommend the triple AFP.

244. The triple panel AFP includes

    (A) Alpha-fetoprotein, estrone, HCG
    (B) Alpha-fetoprotein, estradiol, HCG
    (C) Alpha-fetoprotein, estriol, HCG

245. In counseling this client regarding the AFP testing, you discuss all of the following EXCEPT

    (A) If AFP is high, there is concern for neural tube defects.
    (B) If the AFP is high, there is concern for multiple gestations.
    (C) If the AFP is high, there is concern for Down syndrome.

246. If the AFP is low, you would tell Jamie all the following are true EXCEPT

    (A) If the AFP is low, there is concern for Down syndrome.
    (B) If the AFP is low, there is concern for multiple gestation.
    (C) If the AFP is low, there is concern for incorrect dating.

247. What test would be ordered next if the AFP was high?

    (A) Repeat AFP in 1 week
    (B) Pelvic ultrasound
    (C) Amniocentesis

248. What test would be ordered if the AFP was low?

    (A) Repeat AFP in 1 week
    (B) Pelvic ultrasound
    (C) Amniocentesis

249. Jamie asks about chorionic villus sampling (CVS) testing. Choose the correct statement.

    (A) CVS can be done at 15 weeks' gestation.
    (B) CVS is recommended to be performed prior to 9 weeks' gestation.
    (C) CVS is recommended to be performed between 9 and 10 weeks' gestation.

250. Can CVS screen for neural tube defects?

    (A) Yes
    (B) No; CVS screens for chromosomal abnormalities only but an AFP test is done at the time of the procedure that will screen for NTD.
    (C) No; CVS tests for chromosomal abnormalities only.

Questions 251–253

The following chart depicts fundal height in pregnancy.

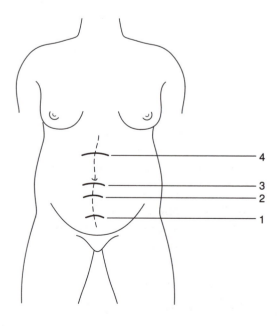

251. What is the appropriate fundal height for a woman at 16 weeks' gestation?

   (A) 1
   (B) 2
   (C) 3

252. Relaxin's role in pregnancy is to

   (A) Relax smooth muscle
   (B) Relax skeletal muscle
   (C) Soften the collagen in articulating joints, especially of the pelvis

253. Normal physiologic respiratory changes that occur in pregnancy include

   (A) Decrease in vital capacity
   (B) Increase in tidal volume
   (C) Decrease in tidal volume

Questions 254–257

A 19-year-old woman at 16 weeks' gestation presents with general malaise, inguinal lymphadenopathy, pain down the top of her legs, difficulty initiating urination, and severe painful vulvar lesions.

254. The most likely diagnosis is

   (A) Chlamydia
   (B) Primary herpes simplex virus (HSV)
   (C) Chancre

255. Prior to 20 weeks' gestation there is

   (A) Increased risk for spontaneous abortion
   (B) Concern for pelvic infection
   (C) Concern of treatment options

256. Acyclovir use in pregnancy is generally

   (A) Recommended
   (B) Not recommended
   (C) Given in labor to prevent neonatal transmission

257. Diagnosis is made by

   (A) Blood typing for HSV I or II

   (B) Virology culture
   (C) DNA probe for multinucleated giant cells

Questions 258–260

As a practitioner you order screening obstetrical ultrasounds on your patients at about 18–20 weeks. The following results are found.

258. An ultrasound at 18 weeks' gestation for screening shows a low-lying placenta. This

   (A) Indicates placenta previa
   (B) May indicate marginal previa
   (C) Usually changes in 6–8 weeks

259. A screening ultrasound at 18 weeks' gestation shows unilateral choriod plexus cyst. This is

   (A) Within normal limits; no need for concern
   (B) An abnormal finding; amnio is recommended
   (C) An abnormal finding; repeat ultrasound is recommended

260. Screening ultrasound shows a fetal ovarian clear cyst. This

   (A) Indicates a need for pediatric consultation
   (B) Usually resolves
   (C) Indicates a need to repeat ultrasound in 6 weeks

Questions 261–264

A woman at 28 weeks' gestation has a 1-hour glucose load test. Her result is 141 mg/dL.

261. This is considered

   (A) Within normal limits
   (B) Abnormal; need 3-hour GTT (glucose tolerance test)
   (C) Abnormal; need fasting blood sugar (FBS) and 2-hour postprandial

262. Risk factors for gestational diabetes include all of the following EXCEPT

   (A) First-degree relative with Type I diabetes
   (B) Prior macrosomic infant
   (C) Obesity >20% of IBW

263. The 3-hour GTT is as follows; FBS, 78; 1 hr, 195; 2 hr, 155; 3 hr, 140; which indicates

   (A) Normal findings—false screen test
   (B) Abnormal with 1 positive value out of 3
   (C) Abnormal with 2 positive values out of 3

264. The next step in managing this client would be

   (A) To do nothing further
   (B) To have a nutrition consult with FBS and 2-hour postprandial
   (C) To have a nutrition consult and initiate insulin with FBS and 2-hr postprandial

Questions 265–269

A woman at 30 weeks' gestation G1 complains of increased vaginal discharge and pressure.

265. You would consider these findings

   (A) Normal
   (B) Indicative of preterm labor (PTL)
   (C) Suspicious for urinary tract infection (UTI)

266. The next step in evaluating this patient would be

   (A) To check cervix for changes
   (B) NST
   (C) Check urine for leukocytes

267. The cervix is posterior, 50%, and 1 cm. Your next step would be

   (A) NST (non-stress test)
   (B) BPP (biophysical profile)
   (C) Reassure the patient of the normal findings

268. What medication is most commonly given for preterm labor (PTL)?

   (A) Terbutaline 2.5 mg every 6 hours
   (B) Nifedipine sc infusion pump
   (C) Terbutaline 10 mg every 6 hours

269. Risk factors for preterm labor inlude all of the following EXCEPT

   (A) Caucasian women
   (B) Multiple gestation
   (C) polyhydramnios

Questions 270–273

A woman at 35 weeks' gestation presents for a routine visit. On Leopold's maneuver, a hard ballotable fetal part is found in the fundus.

270. The fetal position is

   (A) Vertex
   (B) Breech
   (C) Transverse lie

271. At 38 weeks' gestation with the client in labor, the vaginal exam shows posterior chin presentation.

   (A) Expected vaginal delivery
   (B) C-section
   (C) Emergency C-section

272. With vaginal delivery following a cesarean-section (VBAC), the risk is for

   (A) Placenta previa
   (B) Placenta succenturiata
   (C) Uterine rupture

273. The most common tubal ligation procedure is

   (A) Laparoscopy
   (B) Pomeroy
   (C) Bands

Question 274

A woman at 36 weeks' gestation complains of feeling "a little vaginal wetness and some abdominal tightness."

274. The diagnosis of ruptured membranes can be made by

   (A) Ferning on microscopic exam
   (B) A finding of a pH of 5.5 on nitrazine paper
   (C) 2+ WBCs on the wet smear

Questions 275–279

A biophysical is performed and is as follows:

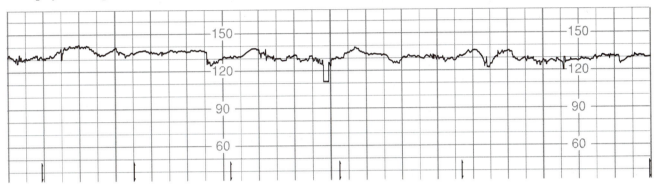

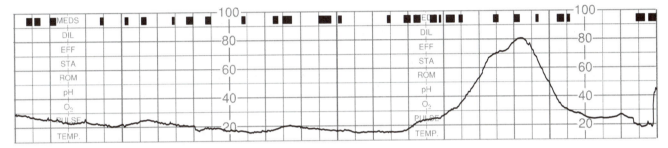

Fetal breathing movements: 1 episode for 35 second duration
Gross body movement: 3 gross movements of body
Fetal tone: Opening and closing of right hand
Amniotic fluid: 1 pocket measuring 2 ½ cm

275.   The significance of one pocket of amniotic fluid measuring 2½ cm is that the patient has
    (A) Normal amniotic fluid
    (B) Oligohydramnios
    (C) Polyhydramnios

276.   Beta-methasone is given for treatment of
    (A) Ruptured membranes
    (B) Premature labor
    (C) Pulmonary hypoplasia

277.   Contractions characteristic of "false labor" are those that
    (A) Become stronger over time
    (B) Increase in strength with walking
    (C) Respond to comfort measures

278.   For Braxton Hicks contractions with the findings on exam of no cervical changes, a pH of 4.0, and no ferning, the next best test to be ordered is

    (A) Urine culture
    (B) Vaginal culture
    (C) Complete blood count (CBC)

279.   The next step in the management of this patient would be

    (A) Repeat NST in 24 hours
    (B) Reevaluate in 1 week
    (C) Perform an L/S ratio or PG determinate

Questions 280–282

A 32-year-old primipara at 36 weeks' gestation complains of increased skin itching with a hive-like rash that started on her belly in her stretch marks and has spread to her arms and legs.

280.   The most likely diagnosis is
    (A) PUPPP (pruritic urticarial papules and plaques of pregnancy)

(B) Pregnancy prurigo

(C) Atopic dermatitis

281. What is an important screening test to order on this client?

(A) Liver function tests (LFT)

(B) Amylase

(C) RPR

282. The correct treatment would be

(A) Oil-based cream such as Eucerin

(B) Water-based cream such as Moisterel

(C) Steroid cream such as Westcort

Questions 283–286

A 27-year-old woman presents with constant and severe low abdominal pain. She had a hysterosalpingogram (HSG) 3 days ago and was premedicated with doxycycline. She denies fever, chills, nausea and vomiting, dysuria, change in bowel pattern, or flank pain. LMP was 14 days ago. Medications include Clomid 50 mg bid days 3–7 (first cycle), prednisone 30 mg po qd, and Ventolin inhaler.

283. The most likely diagnosis is

(A) Mittelschmerz

(B) Pelvic inflamatory disease (PID)

(C) Hyperstimulation

On physical exam her temperature was 98.4°F, abdomen was tender with rebound on right, beta human chorionic gonadotropin (BHCG) < 5, urinalysis negative. The pelvic ulrasound showed top normal uterus, 1.8 cm right ovarian clear cyst, with no free fluid.

284. The most likely diagnosis is

(A) Appendicitis

(B) PID

(C) Hyperstimulation

285. Doxycycline prophalaxis was given for

(A) Mitral valve prolapse (MVP)

(B) PID

(C) Mycoplasm infection

286. Her husband's semen analysis is as follows: volume, 5 mL; pH, 7.2; viscosity, normal; count, 18 million/mL; motility, 73%; morphology, 33%. This result is

(A) Normal

(B) Abnormal; needs to repeat semen analysis.

(C) Abnormal; needs sperm antibody testing

Questions 287–289

Your client and her husband have their first prenatal visit at 9 weeks' gestation. Her ethnic background is Eastern European Ashkenazi and his is English and French Canadian. She also has a history of DES (diethylstilbestrol) esposure in utero.

287. Tay-Sachs testing

(A) Is not necessary

(B) Should be done on the man

(C) Should be done on the woman

288. History of DES exposure in a pregnant woman is of most concern for

(A) Pap smear abnormalities

(B) Cervix incompetency starting at 10 weeks

(C) Cervix incompetency starting at 14 weeks

289. On exam today, a fetal heartbeat is not heard, the client's uterine size is 10–12 weeks, her BP 138/70, and she has severe nausea. The most likely diagnosis is

(A) Blighted ovum

(B) Missed abortion

(C) Molar pregnancy

Questions 290–293

A couple present with concerns about trying to conceive. The woman and her husband are in their 30s and have been trying to become pregnant for 1 year.

290. The nurse practitioner should

(A) Reassure them that this is normal

(B) Encourage them to start IVF

(C) Counsel them about an infertility workup

291. The woman has a family history of an X-linked recessive disorder, which would indicate that

(A) Only females will be affected with the disorder

(B) Only males will be affected with the disorder

(C) Each child regardless of gender has a 1 in 4 chance of being affected

292. The following basal body temperature chart is given to you by the couple for interpretation. You find that

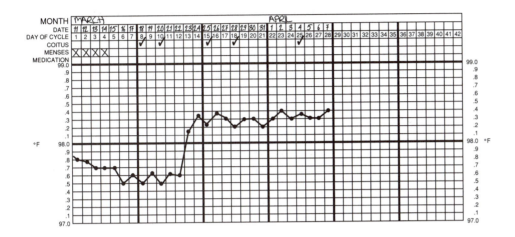

(A) Ovulation occurred on day 13.
(B) Luteal phase defect is present.
(C) Anovulatory cycle is indicated.

293. A postcoital test should be performed

(A) 2–3 hours after sex and within 24 hours after LH surge
(B) 5–6 hours after sex and within 24 hours after LH surge
(C) 3–4 hours after sex and 24 hours before LH surge

Questions 294–298

Casey is a 31-year-old primipara who is 3 days postpartum from a normal spontaneous vaginal delivery. She is currently breast-feeding and has an allergy to penicillin.

294. She telephones the office complaining that her breasts are very swollen and "hard as rock," and her temperature is 99.0°F. The most likely diagnosis is

(A) Breast engorgement
(B) Mastitis
(C) Blocked duct

295. After 2 weeks Casey has right breast demarcation with erythema, tenderness, and a nonfluctuate mass; her temperature is 101°F. The diagnosis is

(A) Mastitis
(B) Breast abscess
(C) Engorgement

296. Management would include

(A) Heat, massage, dicloxacillin 500 mg po q 6h × 10 days
(B) Heat, massage, E-Mycin 500 mg po q 6h × 5 days
(C) Heat, massage, Keflex 500 mg po q 6h × 10 days

297. Casey is concerned about taking 3–4 minutes to experience a let-down. You suggest she

(A) Take oxytocin nasal spray
(B) Perform breast massage
(C) Drink an alcoholic beverage

298. She has a problem with seasonal allergies and would like to know what she can take with breast-feeding. You recommend.

(A) Benadryl
(B) Allegra
(C) Vancenase Nasal Inhaler

Questions 299–301

299. A 57-year-old woman presents with "something falling out of my vagina." Past medical history includes total abdominal hysterectomy (TAH). She takes Premarin 0.625 mg po qd. She has loss of urine with coughing or sneezing. The most likely diagnosis is

(A) Rectocele
(B) Prolapse
(C) Cystocele

300. A client complains that her urine stream is weaker and it takes a long time to urinate, with loss of urine at night. On exam the bladder is palpated above the symphysis pubis. The diagnosis is

(A) Overflow incontinence
(B) Stress incontinence
(C) Urge incontinence

301. A client complains about her urge to urinate after voiding and a history of bedwetting as child. On examination the bladder is not palpable. The diagnosis is

(A) Overflow incontinence
(B) Stress incontinence
(C) Urge incontinence

Answers and Rationales
for Obstetric Cases

188. (C) Hgb A_{1c} test should be ordered along with her prenatal profile to accurately reflect her blood sugars over the last 2 months. This test is useful in evaluating past glucose control. A normal range is 3.5–5.7%. A value greater than 9% represents poor control and increases the risk for congenital abnormalities to 25%. A blood sugar today would be helpful to assess her glycosuria level but the Hgb A_{1c} would be more conclusive. A 24-hour urine collection is necessary on this patient, given her baseline BP in the first trimester. Since it cannot be done on this visit, the patient will have to collect the urine at home.

189. (C) The patient needs to be changed to insulin. Micronase is not used in pregnancy because it can cause congenital abnormalities. The insulin requirement is less in the first trimester but usually increases in the second and third trimester.

190. (C) The Hgb A_{1C} result of 14% indicates that her blood sugars are very out of control. The increase value of the Hgb A_{1c} places her at an increased risk for congenital abnormalities. The Hgb A_{1c} reflects the last 2–3 months of blood sugars. A normal range is less than 9%. FBS in pregnancy should be under 100 and 2-hour postprandial should not exceed 120.

191. (A) As a pre-school teacher she is at risk for the infection with TB, parvovirus antibodies, varicella, and Hepatitis B. A TB skin test should be done at the time of her prenatal visit as well as blood titers for varicella, HBV, and parvovirus. TORCH titer includes testing for toxoplasmosis, rubella, CMV, and herpes. Rubella is part of the prenatal screen done on all prenatal women. Toxoplasmosis would be indicated if she had a cat or did gardening. Herpes titers can have a false positive due to crossover between type 1 and type 2. CMV is an infectious disease that is highly contagious and one that she is at risk for as a preschool teacher, but there is no treatment for the disease and it is presently not recommended to screen women.

192. (A) The correct test to be ordered is a parvovirus IGG and IGM. This test will determine recent exposure versus old infection. The IGM will be elevated in recent exposure and an acute and a convalescent titer would confirm this finding. Parvovirus antibodies would show an old infection but would not be helpful for diagnosis at this point. TORCH does not provide information on Fifth's disease.

193. (A) The test results of parvovirus IGM > 10, IGG < 10 indicate a recent exposure. IGM is the immunoglobulin that rises with infection. The IGG indicates antibodies to the disease and may take up to 3 months to develop. Fifth's disease in adults can present with mild flu-like symptoms with usually no skin rash. Some adults do experience severe joint pain. Past exposure would be evident by > 10 IGG and no exposure would have < 10 in both IGG and IGM.

194. (A) The most likely diagnosis is multiple gestation. A uterus larger than expected for dates (> 4 cm) is the key for the diagnosis. A single intrauterine pregnancy at 7 weeks should be the size of a lemon. An ectopic pregnancy would not present with uterus larger than a date.

195. **(B)** Her risk factors for this diagnosis include all of those except parity. Age does affect the rate of twinning, peaking between 35 and 40 years of age. Race is also a factor in twinning. It is most common in African-Americans, least common in Asians, and intermediate in occurrence in Caucasian women.

196. **(B)** In twin gestation AFP can be done. The maternal serum AFP will average twice the median level for singleton prenancy. The incidence of congenital abnormalities is higher in twin gestation and amniocentesis may also be recommended for this patient given her age of 35 but is not the only test to be ordered. The correct answer is that maternal AFP can be done.

197. **(B)** Prenatal vitamins should have 2 mg of folic acid. Maternal risk with twin gestation includes folic acid deficiency with anemia. One mg of folic acid is recommended for a singleton pregnancy; 400 μg is not enough.

198. **(A)** Dizygotic twins are from 2 ova and 2 sperm. Monozygotic twins are from 1 ova and 1 sperm and are always of the same sex. Dizygotic or fraternal twins may be of the same sex or different sexes.

199. **(C)** Monochorionic and monoamniotic twin gestation is at risk for twin–twin tranfusion due to vascular anastamosis.

200. **(C)** Twin fetal heart rates are usually different and need to be documented. One abnormal pregnancy–induced hypertension (PIH) parameter may be enough to decide upon hospitalization since the client is at risk. Multiple gestation does increase the risk for PTL.

201. **(B)** The MCV is greater than 100. Microcytic is below 82, normocytic is 83–100, and macrocytic is greater than 100. The MCHC is 36%, which is in the normal range of 32–36%. Hypochromic is below 32% and hyperchromic is above 36%.

202. **(A)** Folate level or a B$_{12}$ level would be ordered to differentiate megaloblastic anemia. A ferritin level would be done to evaluate for iron deficiency anemia if the findings were microcytic and hypochromic anemia. TIBC is normally elevated in pregnancy and is not helpful in diagnosis of iron deficiency anemia. Hemaglobin electrophoresis would be done if the MCV was less than 100 or microcytic to evaluate for beta thalassemia.

203. **(C)** Folic acid deficiency is the diagnosis. Megaloblastic anemia during pregnancy is almost always related to folic acid deficiency. The Hgb electrophoresis shows a normal pattern and the ferritin level is within normal levels. Thalassemia or iron deficiency anemia would be a concern if the patient had microcytic not macrocytic anemia.

204. **(B)** A higher dose of folic acid is indicated. Dilantin is a folate antagonist and there is an increased risk to the fetus for facial abnormalities. For this reason it may be recommended to increase folic acid intake to 2 mg.

205. **(C)** Alcohol abuse is related to folic acid deficiency. It is a megaloblastic anemia and can be differentiated from B$_{12}$ deficiency by a low folate level. B$_{12}$ deficiency in pregnant women is related to gastrectomy, Crohn disease, and ileal resection. B$_{12}$ anemia is rare in pregnancy and is related to the lack of intrinsic factor.

206. **(B)** No added iron supplementation is indicated in a woman with β-thalassemia trait. It can be differentiated by a hemoglobin electrophoresis showing an elevated A2 (4–8%) and elevated fetal hemoglobin (1–5%). Microcytic and hypochromic anemia is mild and additional iron supplementation will not correct the anemia. The Hgb concentration is 8–10 g late in second trimester and increases to 9–11 g near term. A prenatal vitamin is given in pregnancy but additional iron is not indicated.

207. **(B)** Mild systolic flow murmur is a normal finding. Diastolic murmurs always require further evaluation with echocardiogram or ECG. Systolic ejection murmurs are very common and related to the increased blood volume in pregnancy.

208. **(C)** O negative with Kell antibodies indicates possible problems for fetal well-being. Atypical antibodies that can cross the placenta and cause fetal hemolysis are Kell, Duffy, Kidd, MNS, Diego, and *P. luthernan.* An ultrasound is done to look for hydrops. Kell antibodies have a 4.5% chance of affecting the fetus.

209. **(A)** If the breast exam reveals a 1-cm firm mass in RUOQ, the next step is a breast ultrasound. There is a concern for breast carcinoma and ultrasound would determine if the mass is solid or cystic. Breast biopsy may be done under local anesthesia.

210. **(B)** Raw eggs are a source of salmonella. Toxoplasmosis is shed in the cat's stool and can be ingested by hand-to-mouth contamination or by inhalation by swallowing the parasite. It is not a concern for inside cats since the virus is from cats eating rodents. Pregnant women should not eat raw meat and should wash hands after handling raw meat. If acute toxoplasmosis infection occurs in the first trimester, elective abortion should be discussed. Toxoplasmosis can cause mental retardation, visual deficits, seizures, hydrocephaly, and hepatosplenomegaly in neonates.

211. **(C)** Placenta previa is not associated with cocaine use in pregnancy. Cocaine use may cause maternal medical complications such as arrhythmias and myocardial infarctions, abruptio placenta (fourfold increase), as well as congenital abnormalities and small size for gestational age. Cocaine causes placental separation by its vasoconstriction and hypertensive effects. Also there is a higher incidence of GU tract abnormalities in babies exposed in utero to cocaine.

212. **(C)** Urine screen for toxicology can be done only with the patient's permission. It cannot be done on urine left for dipstix. The patient has the legal right to refuse urine testing. If the patient agrees to testing, it can be done monthly.

213. **(C)** Intrauterine growth retardation with cocaine use in pregnancy is combined. IUGR is defined as fetal weight below the 10th percentile for gestational age. Asymmetrical growth retardation occurs in the end of the second to third trimester and results in decreased cell size with sparring of the brain cells. Some reasons for asymmetrical growth retardation are maternal diseases such as anemia, hypertension, or renal or vascular disease as well as placenta or cord abnormalities, twins, or postdates. Symmetrical IUGR occurs in the first trimester when fetal growth is related to increase in cell number and is more severe than asymmetrical. The causes can be related to maternal infections such as toxoplasmosis, rubella, or tuberculosis or from fetal abnormalities, first trimester radiation, and poor maternal weight gain. Combined asymmetrical and symmetrical growth retardation is seen with severe malnutrition, alcohol use, and drug use.

214. **(C)** The nicotine patch or gum would not be recommended in pregnancy for a woman who smokes less than a pack of cigarettes a day. With either method the amount of nicotine would exceed her actual present intake. It would be important to try to have the client stop smoking. She may benefit from a smoking-cessation group or use of hypnosis. Smoking in pregnancy is associated with spontaneous abortion, low birth weight, and placental changes that may lead to abruption.

215. **(A)** Alcohol consumption in pregnancy is not recommended. Fetal alcohol syndrome is characterized by prenatal and postnatal growth deficiencies, mental retardation, behavioral problems, and congenital abnormalities. It is associated with an alcohol intake of 3 ounces daily throughout pregnancy. But no safe level for maternal drinking in pregnancy has been established. Studies have demonstrated that binge drinking in pregnancy may carry significant risks for congenital and developmental problems.

216. **(A)** Treat the client with a 10-day course of amoxicillin. Women who have the sickle cell trait are at increased risk for pyelonephritis. All pregnant women should be screened at initial visit for asymptomatic urine infections, since infections of the urinary tract are the most common bacterial infection found in pregnancy. During pregnancy a 10-day course of antibiotics is prescribed because of the 97% cure rate over the 3-day regimen.

217. **(C)** The treatment of choice is TCA. Podophyllin and Condylox are contraindicated in pregnancy as well as 5 fluorouracil cream.

218. **(C)** A pregnant woman with a history of asthma can take Ventolin and Beclovent inhalers. Sometimes oral prednisone is also needed to help asthma symptoms in pregnancy. One third of women will stay the same in pregnancy, one third will be worse, and one third will improve in pregnancy.

219. **(C)** Scopolamine patches are not used in the treatment of hyperemesis gravida. A number of antiemetics may be given to alleviate nausea and vomiting such as Phenergan suppositories and Reglan tablets. With persistent vomiting a workup may be needed to rule out gastroenteritis, pancreatitis, hepatitis, peptic ulcer, and fatty liver of pregnancy. Also, the patient needs to be evaluted for molar pregnancy since a common symptom is severe nausea and vomiting.

220. **(B)** For atypia on a Pap smear at initial exam, the recommendation is to do a colposcopy and repeat the Pap smear at 28 weeks. During pregnancy the transformation zone is exposed due to physiologic eversion. To avoid hemorrhage and rupture of membranes, endocervix curetting is not done. Biopsies are also avoided if possible in pregnancy since the cervix is hyperemic.

221. **(A)** Reassure her that bilateral edema is a common problem that occurs in 80% of pregnancies. It is of concern if the edema is generalized to the face, hands, and feet.

222. **(B)** Order CBC, platelets, chemistry profile with LFT to assess baseline blood work given the findings of BP increased by 25 mm Hg and a significant weight gain with edema in her hands and ankles. PIH can recur in subsequent pregnancy.

223. **(A)** The diagnosis of PIH is confirmed by the blood work. Hemoconcentration causes the hematocrit to rise. Uric acid level, an early blood marker for PIH, is elevated as well as the liver function test indicating hepatic injury. Thrombocytopenia is often present in PIH. Renal function tests are usually within the normal range. Essential hypertension occurs before 15 weeks' gestation and is exhibited by elevated BP without edema, weight gain, or proteinuria. Acute fatty liver disease manifests with nauesea, vomiting, malaise, and jaundice.

224. **(C)** An ophthalmologic exam is indicated for papilledema. Deep tendon reflexes with PIH are brisk and clonus may occur. Orthostatic signs are not present in this patient. Left lateral decubitus blood pressure readings are often done to evaluate the client.

225. **(C)** Jaundice is not a manifestation of PIH. Common symptoms for PIH are headache, visual changes, weight gain, proteinuria, and flu-like symptoms.

226. **(C)** PIH does not occur more frequently in women between the ages of 20 and 30. PIH does occur in teenagers and women 35 or older, as well as primiparas and women with chronic diseases.

227. **(B)** The most likely diagnosis is an ectopic pregnancy given the history of irregular bleeding and severe unilateral pain. Pelvic or abdominal pain is present in over 99% of ectopic pregnancies (DeCherney & Pernoll, 1994). Threatened abortion could be considered a rule-out diagnosis but the correct answer is ectopic. Blighted ovum usually presents with no fetal heart detected on exam, which is then confirmed on ultrasound.

228. **(A)** Risk factors for an ectopic pregnancy do not include birth control pill use. Abdominal or pelvic surgery is a risk factor for ectopic pregnancy secondary to the formation of adhesions. DES exposure is also a risk factor for ectopic pregnancy since it can lead to abnormal tubal structure.

229. **(C)** The correct answer is a transvaginal ultrasound. The minimal discriminatory BHCG level at which an intrauterine sac can be identified by transvaginal ultrasound (TVUS) is 1400 mIU/mL (Montgomery-Rice & Leach, 1993). A repeat quantitative BHCG would be done only after the ultrasound or if the BHCG was initally not greater than 1400 mIU/mL. An MRI would not be indicated for diagnosis of an ectopic preganancy.

230. **(B)** The correct dose is MTX 50 mg/m². The current regimen of methotrexate is a single dose 50 mg/m² intramuscular injection. MTX is given IV as a chemotherapy agent for trophoblastic disease.

231. **(B)** This finding is considered within normal limits and a repeat BHCG is done in 48 hours. Sometimes a slight increase is noted in the BHCG prior to day 7. If there is not a 15% decrease in the BHCG by day 7, a second dose is given. Success rate of this protocol in treating ectopic pregnancy is reported to be 94% (Maiolatesi & Peddicord, 1996).

232. **(B)** She should stop taking the prenatal vitamins since they interact with the MTX protocol. Methotrexate is a folic acid antagonist that interacts with DNA synthesis. Eligibility requirements for this protocol include an unruptured ectopic pregnancy 3.5 cm or less, no active renal or hepatic disease, no evidence of thrombocytopenia or leukopenia, and hemodynamic stability (Maioltesi & Peddicord). It is important to refrain from drinking alcohol and ingesting vitamins with folic acid during MTX therapy.

233. **(C)** The patient's blood bank sample indicates that the patient has received Rhogam. An O negative blood type without antibodies would indicate a need for Rh immunization. Rh sensitivity would be indicated by O negative blood type with a positive indirect Coombs test.

234. **(B)** The diagnosis would be trichomonas and would be confirmed on wet smear by motile trichomonads. The cervix may be friable with noted strawberry patches. Trichomonas does not appear on vaginal culture but may be found on Pap smear samplings. Bacterial vaginosis would show clue cells, lack of WBC, and amine odor. Women can be silent carriers of group B streptococcus infections. The culture for group B streptococcus is taken in the lower vaginal tract to rectum for screening (ACOG, 1992). Symptoms of maternal infection of Group B strep may include dysuria, fever, chills, uterine tenderness (Star, Shannon, Sammons, Lommel, & Gutierrez, 1990).

235. **(A)** The current recommendation would be to treat patient and partner after 12 weeks' gestation with Flagyl tablets. Erythromycin is not effective in the treatment of trichomonas. MetroGel is effective in the treatment of bacterial vaginosis but has not been approved for the treatment of trichomonas. Flagyl is not recommended during the first trimester of pregnancy because its safety has not been established. Trichomonas occurs in about 20–30% of pregnant patients (DeCherney & Pernoll, 1994).

236. **(C)** The correct answer is a false positive. RPR (rapid plasma reagin) and VDRL (venereal disease research lab) are nontreponemal tests. FTA-ABS (fluorescent treponemal antibody absorbed) and MHA-TP (microhemagglutination assay for antibody to *T. pallidum*) are trepomenal tests and remain positive for life regardless of treatment and/or disease activity. False positives can occur secondary to autoimmune disorders such as mononucleosis, malaria, or pneumonia (Cunningham et al, 1997).

237. **(A)** The correct answer is a sTSH. Thyroid function is affected by pregnancy and thyroid disorders are the most common endocrine problems in pregnancy. There is a rise in the thyroxine binding globulin and total thyroxine levels. The free T_4 result may be falsely elevated in pregnancy due to the higher protein levels. The newer and more sensitive TSH assays provide the best test for confirmation of thyroid problems (Reece, Hobbins, Mahoney, & Petrie, 1995).

238. **(B)** Thyroid stimulating immunoglobulins (TSI) may be present in women with active or inactive Graves' disease. These antibodies can cross the placenta and cause fetal or neonatal thyrotoxicosis. If this test is positive an ultrasound is usually done to screen the fetus for thyroid goiter around 30 weeks. Neonatal thyrotoxicosis can be evident at birth with jaundice, tremulousness, diarrhea, tachycardia, goiter, and cardiac failure (Cunningham et al, 1997).

239. **(C)** Ultrasound at 28 weeks' gestation would help evaluate the fetal thyroid gland for goiter or hyperextension of the neck. The fetus can be affected by maternal hormones and antithyroid medication since it crosses the placenta. Fetal growth is assessed throughout the pregnancy to assess for intrauterine growth retardation (IUGR). TSI, specifically maternal immunoglobulin G, can stimulate the fetal thyroid gland (Caldwell, 1996).

240. **(C)** TSI may be an important screening test for this client. She may initially have had Graves' disease and burned out her thyroid gland so that she is now on replacement therapy.

241. **(C)** A PPD should be done unless the client has a history of a prior positive test. The test would be considered positive if the induration was greater than or equal to 10 mm. The patient then would need a chest x-ray after 12 weeks to determine infection or active disease (Cunningham et al, 1997)

242. **(C)** The recommendation would be to begin immunizations since the benefit of receiving vaccine outweighs the risk of contracting the disease. She is considered at high risk given her occupation. HBV infection is spread through sex, blood products, IVDU, and intrauterine or perinatal from mother to baby (Reece, Hobbins, Mahoney, & Petrie, 1995).

243. **(B)** The most conclusive test would be a hemoglobin electrophoresis. A CBC with MCV would help diagnose beta thalassemia or iron deficiency anemia but with a sickle trait the MCV would be normal. The sickledex would screen for sickle trait or disease but not test for beta thalassemia. Persons of African descent have a 1 in 50 chance of having that trait.

244. **(C)** The triple panel AFP includes alpha-fetoprotein, estriol, and HCG. Estradiol is not measured in the triple panel. A low or absent estriol level is of concern for small chromosomal abnormalities carried on the X chromosome.

245. **(C)** The AFP level is low with Down syndrome. The AFP is high for neural tube defects as well as for multiple gestations.

246. **(B)** The AFP level is elevated in multiple gestations. The AFP can be low if pregnancy dating is incorrect and in Down syndrome.

247. **(B)** The first step is accurate dating by pelvic ultrasound because if the dates are off, even by 1 week, this will affect the AFP levels. Amniocentesis would be ordered to rule out chromosomal problems such as Down syndrome if the AFP was low. A repeat AFP may be done but only after the ultrasound since there is some indication that an elevated AFP may indicate placental or preterm problems.

248. **(B)** Pelvic ultrasound should be ordered for dating purposes. A repeat AFP is not ordered if the AFP was initially low. Amniocentesis may be indicated if the dates are correct to rule out genetic disorders.

249. **(C)** CVS is recommended to be performed between 9 and 10 weeks' gestation. CVS is never done at 15 weeks' gestation; however, an early amniocentesis can be done at 15 weeks' gestation. CVS is not done prior to 9 weeks' gestation secondary to the risk of fetal loss and limb abnormalities.

250. **(C)** CVS tests only for chromosomal abnormalities. CVS is done at about 10 weeks' gestation and hence too early for serum AFP testing.

251. **(B)** At 16 weeks' gestation the fundal height should be 4 fingers below the umbilicus. At 20 weeks' gestation the fundus is at the umbilicus.

252. (C) Relaxin is secreted by the corpus luteum of pregnancy, the placenta, and the decidua to soften collagen that affects the articulating surface of the pelvic bones. It relaxes the pubic symphysis and other pelvic joints and may play a role in softening the cervix.

253. (B) Normal respiratory change in pregnancy is a rise in the tidal volume. Dyspnea, a common complaint in pregnancy, is thought to be related to an increase in tidal volume, which then lowers P_{CO_2}, paradoxically causing shortness of breath. The vital capacity is unchanged in pregnancy. The diaphragm rises about 4 cm during pregnancy and the thoracic circumference also increases.

254. (B) Primary HSV (herpes simplex virus). Primary infection usually presents with general malaise, fever, and tender adenopathy. Then the patient may have tingling and then pain at ulcer sites. Chlamydia infections are usually asymptomatic. Chancre is usually a painless, firm ulcer with raised edges and a granulation base. The syphilis ulcer can last up to 6 weeks and then a skin rash can occur.

255. (A) Prior to 20 weeks' gestation, there is a threefold risk in spontaneous abortion with primary HSV. It has been estimated that sexually active women acquire HSV in pregnancy at a rate of 1–2%. Also, primary HSV in pregnancy is associated with an increased rate of asymptomatic shedding of the virus in 10% of women.

256. (B) Acyclovir is currently not recommended for general use in pregnancy. At this time use of acyclovir during pregnancy to prevent viral shedding and neonatal transmission is not recommended for women with a history of recurrence.

257. (B) Diagnosis is made by virology culture. The culture usually is positive for HSV within 48 hours but sometimes is not final until 1 week. Blood typing for HSV type I and type II is usually inaccurate due to a crossover effect. Looking for giant cells on a Pap smear has a poor sensitivity in comparison to a virology culture. It is important to scrape the area first with a spatula and then run the curette over the site. If a HSV lesion is present at time of delivery a C-section may be indicated. Also, if the culture is reported positive after delivery, a pediatric consultation is needed since neonatal infection can occur. Neonatal infection can be skin, eye, and mouth lesions (40%), neurologic symptoms of meningitis (40%), and/or disseminated infection (20%).

258. (C) A low-lying placenta usually changes in 6–8 weeks. Placenta previa would be indicated if the placenta covers the os or part of the os. A repeat ultrasound would be ordered in about 8 weeks to look at the placenta's position.

259. (B) Choriod plexus cyst (CPC) is an abnormal finding and has a 1/300 risk for trisomy 18. The only way to screen for this is by amniocentesis. Ultrasound would not be helpful because even if the CPC resolves the risk for trisomy remains.

260. (C) A fetal ovarian cyst does usually resolve after birth and is probably related to maternal hormones. Ovarian cysts are one of the most common causes of abdominal masses in female neonates. Cysts can increase, decrease, or disappear as well as lead to complications of torsion or rupture. Serial ultrasounds are recommended as well as postnatal scanning for evaluation (Reece et al, 1995).

261. (B) This is considered abnormal—need 3-hour GTT. A 50-g glucose load test is done at 24–28 weeks' gestation with a normal value being less than 140. The 3-hour GTT is the next step.

262. (A) A first-degree relative with Type II diabetes would be a risk factor. A macrosomic infant and obesity are considered risk factors.

263. (B) The 3-hour GTT indicates an abnormal finding with 1 positive value out of 3. FBS should be < 105, 1 hour < 190, 2 hour < 165, 3 hour < 145.

264. **(B)** The next step in managing this client would be a nutrition consult with FBS and 2-hr postprandial. The positive value of 1 out of 3 would indicate this type of intervention. Insulin would be initiated if the FBS was > 130 or if 3 out of 3 values were positive.

265. **(B)** You would consider these findings to be a concern for preterm labor (PTL). Pressure and increased vaginal discharge are common complaints of PTL. Some other symptoms are menstrual-like cramps, abdominal or back pain, urinary frequency, and diarrhea. PTL is defined as labor that occurs after 20 weeks but before 36 weeks. There must be cervical dilatation with intact membranes. PTL is responsible for 75–90% of all neonatal deaths (Cunningham et al, 1997).

266. **(A)** The next step in evaluating this patient would be to check her cervix for changes, since the criteria for PTL are progressive cervical changes over a 30–60 minute interval or a cervix that is 2 cm dilated. A urine culture and NST may also be done as part of the evaluation for this client, but the first step would be to evaluate the cervix.

267. **(A)** Since the cervix is posterior, 50%, and 1 cm, the next step would be a NST to evaluate the client for contractions. If two 30-second contractions occur within 10 minutes over a 20-minute observation along with continuous cervical changes, the diagnosis of PTL can be made.

268. **(A)** Terbutaline 2.5 mg every 6 hours is most commonly given for the management of PTL. Ten mg of terbutaline is an incorrect dose. Nifedipine by mouth, not by infusion pump, is also used for PTL but is more commonly given to women with cervical funneling as opposed to cervical dilatation. Nifedipine is also used for uterine irritability without cervical changes.

269. **(A)** Caucasian women are not as much at risk as African-American women are for PTL. Black race is a risk factor for both PTL and intrauterine growth retardation. The risk is twice that for whites and the cause is unknown. Risk factors for PTL also include multiple gestation and polyhydramnios.

270. **(B)** The fetal position is breech. In breech presentation Leopold's maneuver will reveal a harder, more globular, ballotable fetal part in the fundus. Fetal heart tones are usually heard the loudest above the umbilicus and the patient may report feeling movement low in the abdomen. On transverse lie the uterus looks asymmetrical and wide and you can feel the head and buttocks on the mother's side.

271. **(B)** At 38 weeks' gestation with posterior chin presentation, a cesarean (C-section) may be necessary. Sometimes with posterior chin a vaginal delivery can occur but the important clue is expected. Labor is usually impeded with face presentation since the fetal brow is compressed against the symphysis pubis. Because face presentations are common when there is pelvic inlet contraction, cesarean delivery is frequently done.

272. **(C)** The risk of uterine rupture is low after a previous low transverse incision. Separation of a vertical or classical scar is more likely to occur during VBAC and has an increased risk for uterine perforation. Placenta succenturiata is a placenta lobe separate from the main placenta. This lobe may be retained when the placenta is expelled and lead to postpartum hemorrhage and is not related to VBAC. Placenta previa is also not related to VBAC.

273. **(A)** Laparoscopy is the most common tubal ligation procedure. Electrocautery destroys a large segment of the tube so the failure rate is low. Pomeroy procedure is done as a puerperal tubal sterilization. It is performed by tying absorbable suture material around a loop in the tube and excising above the knuckle of the tube. Bands are placed around the tube and have a higher failure rate.

274. **(A)** A sterile speculum exam is performed and the sample is obtained from the posterior fornix. Amniotic fluid has a pH of 7.0 and turns the nitrazine paper a blue color. A false positive can occur on the nitrazine test if the patient has a bacterial vaginosis, blood, or cervical mucus.

Ferning is performed by touching the sterile Q-tip to the vaginal pool and rubbing it on a glass slide and letting it air dry. False positives can occur if the sample is taken from the cervix instead of the posterior fornix, but the ferning test has an accuracy of 75–98%. Physiologic leukorrhea is an increased amount of normal vaginal discharge that occurs during pregnancy. The wet mount of normal vaginal discharge would not contain 2+ WBCs. This finding may be indicative of a chlamydia infection or yeast vaginitis but would not diagnose ruptured membranes.

275. **(A)** On a biophysical profile the amniotic fluid is considered normal if one pocket measures larger than or equal to 2 cm. Oligohydramnios would be either no amniotic fluid pockets or a pocket less than 1 cm. Oligohydramnios can occur in the third trimester due to post dates or IUGR. Polyhydramnios is an excess quantity of amniotic fluid and is associated with fetal malformation and maternal disease. In polyhydramnios the amniotic fluid index exceeds 25 cm.

276. **(C)** Beta-methasone, a glucocorticoid, has reduced the incidence of neonatal respiratory distress syndrome and is given for pulmonary hypoplasia. Corticosteriods should be given to women with preterm labor before 34 weeks unless infection is suspected or fetal pulmonary maturity is documented. Premature labor is usually treated with tocolysis therapy. Ruptured membranes may be managed by induction depending on gestational age, maternal fever, and period of time.

277. **(C)** Braxton Hicks contractions respond to comfort measures. Painless uterine contractions are felt as tightening or pressure, usually starting at the top of the uterus and pressing down toward the cervix. They usually start at about 28 weeks and can increase in regularity. More than four Braxton Hicks contractions in an hour is a sign of premature labor. These "false contractions" usually disappear with walking or exercise, whereas true labor contractions increase in strength with walking and become stronger over time.

278. **(A)** The next best test to be ordered is a urine culture. As the uterus enlarges, the bladder is displaced upward and flattened in the anterior–posterior position. Clinically the patient may present with urinary frequency, a common complaint in pregnancy. Often women have Braxton Hicks contractions due to the position of the bladder and the inability to empty it completely. A urine culture and sensitivity should be done. The drugs of choice in the treatment of cystitis would be amoxicillin, Macrodantin, or cephalosporins for 10 days. A CBC would be ordered for the management of clients with ruptured membranes but not for this case study. A vaginal culture is performed to test for group B beta streptococcus infections and vaginitis. Women can be streptococcus carriers and not exhibit any unusual symptoms. Clients with yeast vaginitis in pregnancy usually have vaginal itching, not Braxton Hicks contractions.

279. **(B)** Reevaluate the client in 1 week. The biophysical is 8/10 score. Two points each for fetal breathing, gross body movements, fetal tone, and amniotic fluid. The NST is non-reactive. There are no accelerations of greater than or equal to 15 bpm for at least 15 seconds' duration. According to Manning the risk of fetal asphyxia is extremely rare and intervention is not indicated. NST has a high false positive rate due to sleep–wake cycles of the fetus, maternal ingestion of fluids and food, and gestational age.

280. **(A)** Pruritic urticarial papules and plaques of pregnancy (PUPPP) begins in the third trimester and is characterized by hive-like patches that start in the stretch marks and can spread over abdomen, thighs, and extremities but never on the face. PUPPP is usually seen in primiparas and recurrence in subsequent pregnancies is rare. Pregnancy prurigo usually starts on the extremities and begins in the second trimester. Atopic dermatitis can occur in pregnancy but usually the patient has a prior history.

281. **(A)** Liver function tests will rule out liver disease. Amylase would help evaluate pancreatitis but is not indicated in this case study. RPR would screen for syphilis but is not the concern since the rash is not on the palms.

282. **(C)** Mild potency steroid cream such as West-cort is the choice in the management of PUPPP. An oil-based cream may be used in the treatment of atopic dermatitis. A water-based cream is sometimes used in the treatment of pregnancy prurigo.

283. **(C)** Hyperstimulation occurs most commonly in the first cycle of Clomid. Clients often persent with abdominal pain. It is important not to do a pelvic exam on a client with hyperstimulation since it may cause rupture of the follicle. Hyperstimulation occurs in 2% of population during initial dose. Clomid acts as antiestrogen to provoke a response from the pituitary. It works in inducing ovulation in about 70% of women who are producing estrogen but have irregular cycles. A follicle is usually 3 cm in size but with hyperstimulation the follicle can be 8–9 cm in size. Common side effects of clomiphene include hot flashes, depression, and/or bloating.

284. **(B)** PID is likely since she has recently had a HSG and the ultrasound showed no indication of appendicitis. Ultrasound is about 91–95% accurate in the diagnosis of appendicitis and can allow differentiation between acute appendix and gangrenous/perforated appendix (DeCherney & Pernoll, 1994). The client is on prednisone 30 mg daily for asthma, which may give a false temperature reading. HSG is done by injecting dye into the uterus using a catheter. Salpingitis can occur in about 1–3% of women. This test is contraindicated in women with an adnexal mass or allergy to iodine or radiocontrast dye. Hyperstimulation would be evident on ultrasound by the findings of a follicle 8–9 cm in size.

285. **(B)** Doxycycline was given for prophylaxis for PID. Salpingitis can occur in about 1–3% of women following a HSG procedure. Mitral valve prolapse prophylaxis is given to prevent endocarditis and is usually pencillin or amoxicillin. Mycoplasma infections are treated with doxycycline, but the concern is salpingitis.

286. **(B)** The semen analysis is abnormal and needs to be repeated. The count is below normal (20–500 million), motility is within normal (50–100%), morphology is abnormal (40–100%), and the pH is normal (7.2–7.8). According to DeCherney and Pernoll (1994) a repeat semen analysis should be done 72 days after initial testing to provide accurate information. Sperm antibody testing would be done if the postcoital testing was abnormal or the second semen analysis showed poor results.

287. **(B)** Tay-Sachs testing should be done on the man. If he is not a carrier, no further testing is necessary. Tay-Sachs disease is autosomal recessive. You need both parents to be carriers to have a child affected by the disease. The chance for each offspring is 1 out of 4. Two out of four children will be carriers if both parents are carriers. Tay-Sachs testing is not done on the pregnant woman because it can be inconclusive.

288. **(C)** History of diethylstilbestrol (DES) exposure in a pregnant woman is of most concern for cervical incompetency starting at 14 weeks. Cervix incompetency can occur when the fetus applies pressure to the cervix and typically occurs after 10 weeks. Pap smear abnomalities are a concern for DES exposure, especially clear cell adenocarcinoma, but the best answer is cervix incompetency.

289. **(C)** The most likely diagnosis is molar pregnancy. The symptoms are elevated blood presssure, severe nausea and vomiting, uterine size larger than dates, and no fetal heartbeat. An ultrasound would confirm the findings and usually shows a snow-storm pattern. Hydatiform mole needs to be followed closely after the dilatation and evacuation (D&E) with serial beta human chorionic gonadotropins (BHCGs). Most of the time there is a 14-week decline of BHCG to zero (DeCherney & Pernoll, 1994) and then the BHCG is repeated monthly until 1 year.

290. **(C)** Evaluation is recommended since the couple is in their 30s and have not conceived after 1 year of trying to become pregnant. The cause of infertility can be identified in most couples with ⅓ being male factor, ⅓ female factor, and

⅓ combination of male and female factors. The best response would be to educate and counsel the couple about the infertility workup. The first step is not IVF.

291. **(B)** Only males can be affected by a recessive X-linked disorder. Some examples of X-linked disorders are color-blindness, hemophilia A, and Duchenne muscular dystrophy. Half of the male offspring or sons of a carrier mother will be affected with the disorder. The daughters of the carrier mother may become carriers of the disorder. The males are affected because they have only one X-chromosome, inherited from the mother. The Y chromosome is genetically linked to the father.

292. **(A)** Ovulation occurred on day 13, as indicated by the rise in temperature for 2 days after the LH surge. The temperature is lower in the first part of the cycle with a rise of 0.4–0.6°F between a 24-hour reading with ovulation. If the client is pregnant, the temperature would rise and stay elevated. It is important to instruct the patient she must stay in bed for a minimum of 4 hours before taking her temperature. A luteal phase defect would be indicated if the basal body temperature rise lasted less than 10 days. An anovulatory cycle would have erratic temperature readings with no clear delineation between the follicular and luteal phase.

293. **(A)** The optimum time for a postcoital test is 2–3 hours after sex and within 24 hours of LH surge. This test looks at sperm motility and cervical mucus. LH surge occurs within 24 hours of ovulation. A normal postcoital test shows clear mucus with a spinnbarkeit of greater than 10 cm. Ferning would be visible under microscopic exam and confirm ovulation. Also, in a normal postcoital test, the practitioner would see 5–10 motile sperm swimming across the slide under high-power field.

294. **(A)** Breast engorgement typically occurs when the milk comes in around day 3. Mastitis rarely occurs before the fifth postpartum day and usually presents between the second and fourth weeks. A blocked duct would occur at one site on the breast.

295. **(A)** Mastitis is differentiated from engorgement by the onset of fever and the breast exam findings of erythema, tenderness, and mass. Fluctuation, if present, is a wavy impulse felt on palpation and would indicate a breast abscess.

296. **(C)** Management includes heat, massage, and Keflex 500 mg po q6h × 10 days. Dicloxacillin would not be given to a penicillin-allergic patient. While E-Mycin is indicated for the most common organism (*Staphylococcus aureus*) that causes mastitis, its course of treatment—only 5 days—is not sufficient and relapse may occur. The best choice is Keflex 500 mg.

297. **(B)** Breast massage is the best choice to help let-down. Oxytocin nasal spray was used to help decrease let-down time but is no longer on the market. The use of an alchoholic beverage may not be acceptable to the client as a choice. In addition, alchohol can act as a diuretic and affect the milk supply.

298. **(C)** For seasonal allergies while breast-feeding, the best choice is Vancenase Nasal Inhaler, since it is not absorbed systemically. Benadryl is not recommended while breast-feeding since it can affect neonates. Allegra is not recommended since it is a new medication with limited information regarding safe use in pregnancy and/or breast-feeding.

299. **(C)** Cystocele is indicated since she had a complete hysterectomy. Cystocele is a soft mass that can bulge into the vagina and distend the introitus. Symptoms are aggravated by prolonged standing, coughing, sneezing, or straining. Urinary incontinence is the most common symptom of cystocele. Management is done by pessary, Kegel exercises, and/or surgery. Prolapse refers to a falling down of the pelvic organs. A rectocele is a soft mass bulging into the lower half of the vaginal wall. Women complain of difficulty with bowel movments and may need to insert a finger into the vagina to help push out stool.

300. **(A)** With overflow incontinence, the urethra is narrowed by scar tissue or a prolapsed organ such as benign prostatic hyperplasia (BPH) or retroverted uterus in pregnancy, and the bladder never empties completely. The pressure becomes so great that the external spincter cannot stay closed. The type of treatment depends upon the cause of the incontinence. It may be surgery, pessary, medications such as alpha-adrenolytic agents, or self-catheterizations.

301. **(C)** Urge incontinence is caused by an overly sensitive bladder, which feels full even when it contains a small amount of urine. Urge incontinence can be sensory or motor related. Sensory incontinence occurs in a stable bladder and is not due to excessive descent of the urethra and bladder. Common causes are urine infection, neoplasia, and foreign bodies, as well as psychological and neurogenic factors. Motor urge incontinence is the result of an unstable bladder due to involuntary contractions. Treatment again depends upon the cause and consists of medication such as anticholinergics for bladder spasms, antibiotics, estrogen therapy, surgery, and bladder training exercises.

III

Primary Care

Primary Care Cases and Questions

Questions 302–305

The following questions relate to the diagram of the chest.

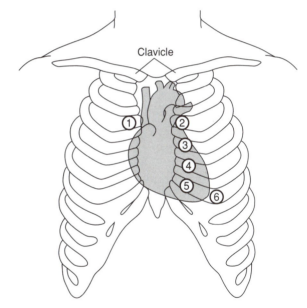

Figure 302

302. Where on the chest wall is S_1 softer than S_2?

(A) 1
(B) 6
(C) 3

303. Where on the chest wall is S_1 usually louder than S_2?

(A) 2
(B) 4
(C) 5

304. The mitral valve sounds are best heard at what position?

(A) 2
(B) 3
(C) 6

305. By asking the client to sit up, lean forward, exhale completely, and stop breathing in expiration and then listening with the diaphragm of the stethoscope at the left sternal border, the clinician is evaluating

(A) Mitral murmurs
(B) Aortic murmurs
(C) Mitral valve prolapse

Questions 306–310

306. A teenage girl reveals a positive family history of smoking by both parents. Her major risk factor associated with an increased likelihood of becoming a chronic cigarette smoker is

(A) Female gender
(B) Her age
(C) Passive aggressive personality profile

307. The most effective primary prevention strategy for the nurse practitioner to implement for teen smoking prevention would be to

(A) Teach specific skills for resisting social pressure
(B) Refer her to a smoking-cessation group
(C) Instill fear in her

308. The greatest *immediate* benefit of smoking cessation is the reduction in

    (A) Lung cancer
    (B) Cardiovascular risk
    (C) Weight gain

309. You would expect the above client's pulmonary function tests to be

    (A) Abnormal
    (B) Normal
    (C) Generally normal unless respiratory illness is present

310. The leading cancer death in women is _____ cancer.

    (A) Breast
    (B) Lung
    (C) Cervical

Questions 311–313

A young college student has recurring trouble associated with drinking alcohol. Her screening for problem drinking reveals chronic fatigue, difficulty concentrating, frequent hangovers, and mood swings. She is having difficulty in school because of chronic absenteeism.

311. You would advise her that

    (A) You consider her drinking behavior as hazardous
    (B) Binge drinking is part of campus life
    (C) She has a poor prognosis for recovery

312. Based on your knowledge of alcohol abuse with heavy drinkers, you know the amount of drinking is _____ by the patient.

    (A) Underestimated
    (B) Overestimated
    (C) Reported accurately

313. The most popular screening test for alcohol abuse and dependence in the primary care setting is the

    (A) MAST (Michigan Alcoholism Screening Test)
    (B) CAGE questionnaire
    (C) AUDIT (Alcohol Use Disorders Identification Test)

Questions 314–316

A 19-year-old female presents with headaches that last most of the day. Her headaches are preceded by an episode of seeing a gleam of light in the right visual field for several minutes, which gradually resolves and is followed by a throbbing right-sided headache. Her headache is associated with pain behind her eyes, which after several hours spreads over her entire head; she also feels nauseated. The patient's mother has migraine headaches.

314. Your most likely diagnosis for the above client would be

    (A) Temporal ateritis
    (B) Tension headache
    (C) Migraine headache

315. Frequent symptoms accompanying migraine headaches are nausea, vomiting, and

    (A) Constipation
    (B) Photophobia
    (C) Forgetfulness

316. The agent of choice for moderate and severe attacks in the pharmacologic treatment of migraines is

    (A) Simple analgesics
    (B) Ergot-containing drugs
    (C) Propranolol

Question 317

A 32-year-old graduate student presents with recurrent headache that feels "like a band over the top of my head." The headaches occur almost daily in the late afternoon and last for several hours when in school. She denies headache while on vacation or on weekends. She denies nausea or vomiting and has no family history of migraines. Physical exam is unremarkable except for cervical tenderness.

317. You suspect

    (A) Transient ischemic attacks (TIAs)
    (B) Cluster headache
    (C) Tension headache

Questions 318–320

Anne comes into your office with a complaint of facial acne. She is a 35-year-old woman with no prior history of skin eruptions. She has tried several over-the-counter products and oral antibiotics without success. She is taking multivitamins and Lopressor for high blood pressure. Her lipid profile is: total cholesterol, 200; HDL, 52; and LDL, 120. Her triglyceride level is normal. She uses withdrawal for birth control. She adds that she is depressed about her skin condition.

318. The clinician diagnoses her with cystic acne. She prescribes Accutane (13 *cis*-retinoic acid). What is the most significant concern for Anne?

   (A) Teratogenic effects
   (B) Lipid elevation
   (C) Reduced night vision

319. What screening tests should be ordered prior to initiation of treatment and at monthly intervals during treatment?

   (A) Triglycerides, cholesterol, and glucose
   (B) Triglycerides, cholesterol, and liver enzymes
   (C) Complete blood count, triglycerides, and cholesterol

320. What side effects occur frequently with use of Accutane?

   (A) Dry skin and eyes
   (B) Leukepenia
   (C) Reduced night vision

Questions 321–324

A young woman is planning to conceive within the next year and is seeking advice for a healthy outcome.

321. You would advise her that preconception care is an appropriate primary prevention strategy and should begin

   (A) Within 1 year of planning pregnancy
   (B) As soon as she misses a period
   (C) At 12 weeks' gestatation

322. In discussing the rationale for preconception care to the client, you explain that organogenesis occurs

   (A) Between day 32 and day 84 after fertilization
   (B) Between day 17 and day 56 after fertilization
   (C) Between day 29 and day 96 after fertilization

323. The goal of preconception care is to

   (A) Assist the patient to achieve her ideal body weight prior to conception
   (B) Maximize the health of the woman and the health of her potential infant
   (C) Begin teaching the process of childbirth as early as possible

324. You would advise her to take _____ folic acid per day for reducing the risk of neural-tube-defect.

   (A) 0.4 mg
   (B) 1.4 mg
   (C) 4.4 mg

Questions 325–329

Alison is in for her initial visit. She wants to discuss future pregnancy plans. She is a 35-year-old G1 P1 who has rheumatoid arthritis (RA). She was diagnosed 6 months ago after seeking evaluation for increasing joint pain and stiffness. She presently controls her symptoms with aspirin, local heat, exercise, and adequate sleep and rest.

325. Which is the typical onset pattern of rheumatoid arthritis?

   (A) Insidious onset with slow, progressive development of symptoms over weeks to months
   (B) Fatigue upon waking
   (C) Initial redness overlying joints

326. What statement is true concerning pregnancy and its effect on patients with rheumatoid arthritis?

   (A) Exacerbation of inflammatory symptoms
   (B) Remission of symptoms that recur postpartum
   (C) No effect on the course of disease

327. Alison is taking aspirin for treatment of RA. What is the earliest manifestation of ASA toxicity?

   (A) Gastrointestinal bleeding
   (B) Tinnitus or mild deafness
   (C) Severe headaches and visual changes

328. What is true about the interpretation of rheumatoid factor?

   (A) RF of 1:20 is strongly positive and indicative of an acute exacerbation.
   (B) RF is highly sensitive at the onset of the disease.
   (C) RF can be positive in a normal population in adults greater than 50 years of age.

329. Criteria for diagnosis of RA must include which of the following?

   (A) Morning stiffness
   (B) Persistent swelling of the joints for longer than 6 weeks
   (C) Difficult weight bearing on the affected joints

Questions 330–333

A 28-year-old woman complains of having had 3–4 weeks of sleep problems, lack of energy, loss of weight, feeling unhappy, inability to concentrate, as well as feeling sad and under a lot of stress.

330. The possible diagnosis is

   (A) Premenstrual syndrome (PMS)
   (B) Major clinical depression
   (C) Thyroid problems

331. Risk factors for depression include all the following EXCEPT

   (A) Family history
   (B) Gender
   (C) Marital status

332. A pregnant woman is on Prozac for clinical depression and asks you if she should continue its use during pregnancy. You respond,

   (A) Yes, it is a category B drug whose benefits outweigh the risk.

   (B) No, it is not recommended during pregnancy and you must wean off the medication.
   (C) No, it is not recommended in pregnancy and you must stop immediately.

333. Starting 5 days postpartum, a woman experiences insomnia and weepiness lasting a few hours every day. The most likely diagnosis is

   (A) Maternity blues
   (B) Postpartum depression
   (C) Anxiety disorder

Question 334–338

A 30-year-old woman is on oral antiinflammatory corticosteroids and is thinking of starting oral contraceptives.

334. The nurse practitioner (NP) needs to know whether oral corticosteroids and oral contraceptives have a drug interaction. Oral contraceptives

   (A) Increase the effect of corticosteroids
   (B) Decrease the effect of corticosteroids
   (C) Do not have a significant effect on corticosteroids

335. On physical exam of the client, you palpate an enlarged thyroid gland. As part of her workup you order thyroid function studies. The NP should know that oral contraceptives can

   (A) Increase free thyroxin
   (B) Elevate thyroid-binding globulin (TBG)
   (C) Decrease TBG

336. The client asks you about taking vitamin C supplements while on oral contraceptives to improve her immune function. She should be advised that vitamin C at doses of 1 g or more per day

   (A) Decreases the amount of ethinyl estradiol absorbed
   (B) Increases the amount of ethinyl estradiol absorbed
   (C) Has an adverse effect on the progestin

337. For the client on anticonvulsants, the NP should use which of the following oral contraceptives?

(A) The lowest dose oral contraceptive possible, such as 20 µg of ethinyl estradiol
(B) A higher dose oral contraceptive with 50 µg ethinyl estradiol
(C) Avoid estrogen completely and use a progestin-only minipill

338. Patients on oral contraceptives should be advised of the following when taking antibiotics.

(A) Antibiotic use will lead to decrease in the efficacy of oral contraceptives.
(B) There is no firm evidence of contraceptive failure in oral contraceptive users on antibiotics.
(C) Clients who are on oral contraceptives should not take antibiotics.

Questions 339–341

Dot is a 37-year-old patient who has an appointment for her annual examination. She is a healthy woman without chronic illness or complaints. She has a history of basal cell carcinoma and childhood sunburns. She admits to direct sun exposure but applies sunscreen when she goes to the beach. She would like you to examine her skin for any atypical lesions. She has not seen her dermatologist for 2 years.

339. The clinician is performing a skin examination. What characteristics do *not* increase the risk of melanoma?

(A) The patient has fair skin and history of childhood sunburns.
(B) The patient uses Accutane (isotretinoin) as recommended by her dermatologist.
(C) The patient's lesions are larger than 6 mm in size.

340. The clinician identifies a scaly, circular lesion with a thread-like border that is 7 mm in diameter. What would be the next step in evaluating this patient?

(A) Treat with a steroid cream to resolve contact dermatitis.
(B) Perform a skin biopsy.
(C) Observe and reevaluate in 3 months.

341. What statement is true concerning non-melanoma skin cancers?

(A) Significant risk factors are cumulative sun exposure, skin color, and age.
(B) Basal cell carcinoma commonly metastasizes at the rate of 3–10% of all lesions.
(C) The majority of nonmelanoma skin cancers occur on the trunk.

Questions 342–346

Ricky is a 38-year-old G0 P0 who has an appointment for her annual examination. She is reviewing her medical history and has questions about immunizations and appropriate intervals and preventive vaccines. She is a healthy woman with allergies to wheat and eggs. She has recently been notified of a co-worker's diagnosis of hepatitis A.

342. Modern vaccines are highly purified and allergic reactions are rare. History of a severe adverse reaction is a contraindication to further use. Patients must be screened for food and medication allergies prior to inoculation. Ricky can receive which of the following vaccines?

(A) Influenza vaccine
(B) Yellow fever vaccine
(C) Hepatitis vaccine

343. Ricky has concerns about her co-worker's diagnosis of hepatitis A. They have recently started an intimate relationship. What would be an appropriate step to decrease her risk of acquiring this virus?

(A) Hepatitis A vaccine
(B) Immune globulin
(C) Instruct the patient in precautions and prevention as no vaccine is available

344. What facts are true concerning tetanus vaccine?

(A) Majority of cases of tetanus occur in young children not fully immunized.
(B) Tetanus usually follows animal bites and penetrating wounds.
(C) Tetanus boosters should be given at the time of any penetrating wound regardless of last immunization.

345. Which statement is true concerning influenza vaccine?

(A) Mild respiratory infections are a contraindication to injection.
(B) The vaccine is 70–80% effective with lower rates of efficacy in elderly and debilitated persons.
(C) The recommended polyvalent should contain type A and B antibodies of strains expected in the upcoming season.

346. MMR vaccine has just been given to your patient following a negative rubella titre. What is the most common side effect of this vaccine?

(A) Fever
(B) Rash
(C) Arthralgias 1–3 weeks following immunization

Questions 347–354

Althea is a 38-year-old woman who has an appointment for an acute care visit. The patient claims to be in good health without chronic illness or use of regular medications. She is currently complaining of persistent fatigue, flu-like symptoms, and nausea. She also notes constant abdominal discomfort but denies changes in bowel or bladder habits. She denies vaginal discharge, dysuria, and dyspareunia. She has been in a monogamous relationship for 2 years. Physical exam reveals a tender, palpable liver.

347. The clinician orders a urinalysis and culture. What evidence may alert the clinician to a diagnosis of hepatitis?

(A) Proteinuria
(B) Bilirubinuria
(C) Hematuria

348. What is the most common type of hepatitis?

(A) Hepatitis A
(B) Hepatitis B
(C) Hepatitis C

349. Clinical symptoms of hepatitis subtypes are similar. At what stage are patients most likely to seek medical attention?

(A) Fatigue, nausea, and flu-like symptoms
(B) Anorexia, abdominal discomfort, skin rash, and arthralgias
(C) Jaundice, pruritus, and dark urine

350. The clinician orders a liver profile. What value generally rises before evidence of jaundice?

(A) Alkaline phosphatase
(B) Aminotransferases
(C) Albumin

351. A sudden rapid fall in serum aminotransferases from a high peak to normal in less than 1 week can be an indication of

(A) Increased risk of chronic hepatitis
(B) Beginning of recovery phase
(C) Fulminant hepatitis with risk of liver necrosis

352. Althea returns for follow-up visits every 2 weeks to monitor clinical symptoms and lab values. Her surface antigen is measured after 6 months and is positive. What is the next step in management for this patient?

(A) Return in 6 months for repeat testing.
(B) Refer to hepatologist for management of chronic hepatitis.
(C) Counsel patient that her surface antigen will be positive for several months.

353. Alcoholic hepatitis and viral hepatitis may have similar clinical presentations such as anorexia, fatigue, jaundice, and hepatomegaly. Patients with alcoholic hepatitis are more likely to have which of the following?

(A) Elevated temperature, leukocytosis
(B) Elevated serum aminotransferases
(C) Milder illness as compared to viral hepatitis

354. Elevated serum aminotransferases and alkaline phosphatase are occasionally found in patients without liver disease. What test would confirm hepatic involvement?

(A) Elevated serum 5'-nucleotidase
(B) Elevated creatine kinase
(C) Elevated bilirubin

Questions 355–358

Amanda is a 39-year-old woman who presents at your practice for her annual examination. She admits to a change in bowel habits with an increase in constipation. She also complains of abdominal discomfort, bloating, and blood in her stool. She denies any significant dietary changes. She takes Synthroid for hypothyroidism. She has no allergies to medications and has no other complaints. She has a history of ulcerative colitis, which is controlled with diet and stress-reduction techniques. She had two rectal polyps removed 3 years ago and has annual rectal exams by stool guaiacs for follow-up.

355. The clinician performs a physical exam on the patient. Her abdomen is soft and nontender without hepatomegaly. Bowel sounds are decreased. Her stool guaiac is positive, but no rectal masses are detected on exam. What would be the next step in her evaluation?

   (A) Send the patient home with a stool guaiac kit to test 3 consecutive stools
   (B) Proctosigmoidoscopy
   (C) Abdominal ultrasound

356. What history is *not* significant in increasing the risk of colon cancer for this patient?

   (A) Ulcerative colitis
   (B) Colonic polyps
   (C) Cigarette smoking of 5 years' duration

357. What causes a false-negative result in occult blood screening?

   (A) Iron compounds
   (B) High doses of vitamin C
   (C) Peroxidase-rich foods

358. Colonic polyps are associated with colon cancer. What statement is true concerning polyps?

   (A) The majority of colon cancers (excluding those associated with ulcerative colitis) originate from benign epithelial tumors.
   (B) Polyps are found exclusively in the rectosigmoid region.
   (C) Polyps are commonly identified in clusters and complete removal of lesions results in rare recurrence.

Questions 359–361

Joan P. presents at the office for an annual examination. As the clinician elicits the history she finds that the patient has a family history of melanoma and a personal history of sunburn during childhood. The patient admits to tanning during the summer months and occasionally using tanning salons during the winter. Her physical examination reveals multiple nevi distributed over her trunk, extremities, and face. The clinician uses a magnifying lens and notes the color, size, and borders of the lesions. She recommends that Joan see a dermatologist for skin cancer screening.

359. The familial atypical mole and melanoma syndrome (FAMM) is a significant risk factor in skin cancer screening. Which characteristics best describe this syndrome?

   (A) Individuals begin to develop atypical lesions at puberty and throughout life.
   (B) Family history may include melanoma.
   (C) The lifetime risk of melanoma approaches 50%.

360. What clinical characteristic is *not* associated with atypical or dysplastic nevi?

   (A) Round tan to dark-colored lesions with sharply defined borders
   (B) Large macular or papular lesions greater than 6 mm in size
   (C) Irregular borders with variable degrees of brown, tan, black, red, and/or blue color

361. What counseling would you give to this patient?

   (A) Annual screening by a clinician to observe for atypical lesion development that may be associated with melanoma
   (B) Daily use of sunscreen on exposed skin surfaces and avoidance of direct, prolonged sun exposure during peak hours
   (C) Self-examination of skin every 6 months

Questions 362–374

Babs presents at your office for her annual exam. She is a 40-year-old G2 P2 with no significant history of chronic illness, gynecologic abnormalities, or current medications. She has noted some dry skin, hair loss, lack of energy, and three missed periods over the last 6 months. She has a low-fat, high-fiber diet, runs 3–4 miles per day, and denies significant stress. She complains of constipation despite her high-fiber diet and regular exercise. Her physical examination is normal with a 4-lb weight gain since her last visit. Her thyroid is smooth and palpable, vital signs are stable, and deep tendon reflexes are delayed in their relaxation phase. A mental status exam is normal. The thyroid profile reveals an elevated TSH, low T_4, and low FTI.

362. What is the single most important measurement of clinical evaluation of thyroid disease?

   (A) T_3
   (B) TSH
   (C) T_4

363. The free T_4 is estimated by separate measurements of non-protein-bound T_4 and total T_4. When is the measurement of free T_4 problematic in interpretation? With

   (A) Pregnancy
   (B) Estrogen therapy
   (C) Chronic liver disease

364. What finding(s) is usually diagnostic of Graves' disease and absent in patients with toxic nodular goiter?

   (A) Asymmetrical enlargement of the thyroid gland
   (B) A bruit over the thyroid gland
   (C) Cardiovascular findings including sinus tachycardia, systolic flow murmurs, and wide pulse pressure

365. Babs complained of several symptoms associated with hypothyroidism. What symptoms point to a *hyperthyroid* state?

   (A) Cold intolerance, muscle aches, fatigue, lethargy, and increased sleep requirement
   (B) Dry, scaling skin, hair loss, facial puffiness
   (C) Weight loss, heat intolerance, sweats, palpitations, and anxiety

366. Babs is currently receiving replacement therapy but her medical records are unavailable

and history is vague. the next step in her management would be:

   (A) Continue current therapy
   (B) Increase the dose of thyroid and recheck TSH and T_4 in 1 month
   (C) Discontinue the current therapy and recheck free T_4 and TSH in 5 weeks

367. How long will it take to restore Babs to a normal metabolic state?

   (A) 6–8 weeks
   (B) Several months
   (C) 4 weeks

368. What lab test is most cost effective in following the titration phase of thyroid replacement therapy?

   (A) T_3
   (B) T_4
   (C) TSH

369. At what point do you perform lab tests following a dosage change?

   (A) 4 weeks
   (B) 6–8 weeks
   (C) 12 weeks

370. After the endpoint of therapy is reached with TSH and T_4 within normal ranges, how often would you perform thyroid function tests?

   (A) Every 6 months
   (B) Annually
   (C) Every 6 weeks

371. What symptoms are *not* associated with Graves' disease?

   (A) Low-pitched voice
   (B) Lid retraction with increased scleral visibility above and below the iris, infrequent blinking, and extraocular muscle weakness
   (C) Hand tremor

372. One of the most frequent abnormalities of the thyroid gland is the presence of a palpable nodule. What test is the first step necessary in ruling out malignancy?

(A) Scintiscan
(B) Needle biopsy
(C) Excisional biopsy

373. What type of nodule is associated with the highest risk of cancer?

(A) Hot nodule
(B) Cold nodule
(C) Multinodular goiter

374. Which type of thyroid cancer is highly aggressive and invasive?

(A) Follicular carcinoma
(B) Anaplastic carcinoma
(C) Medullary carcinoma

Questions 375–378

Margot is a 42-year-old G0 P0 who at her initial examination claims to be in good health without chronic illness or use of regular medications. She has not had a Pap smear for 5 years. She is in a long-term monogamous relationship with a woman partner. They have recently adopted a 1 year-old daughter from China. Her partner's mother lives with them as she has debilitating arthritis and limited mobility. She admits to considerable stress as she adapts to motherhood and sharing the care of a dependent elder.

375. What is the most serious health risk for lesbians?

(A) Substance abuse
(B) Avoidance of regular health care visits
(C) Depression

376. Which statement is true concerning sexually transmitted disease among lesbians?

(A) Cervical dysplasia and cancer are rarely reported in lesbian population populations.
(B) The incidence of gonorrhea, chlamydia, and syphilis is low among lesbians.
(C) Human papilloma virus cannot be transmitted between women during sexual activity without penetration.

377. What is true about breast cancer risk and lesbians?

(A) Nulliparity and absence of lactation increase the risk of breast cancer for this group of women.
(B) Research shows that lesbians are at greater risk for breast cancer compared to heterosexual women.
(C) No data or studies are available that show that lesbian sexual orientation increases or decreases breast cancer risk.

378. Which subgroup of lesbians is at particular risk for psychological problems?

(A) Women greater than age 65
(B) Women still in the closet about sexual identity
(C) Youths and teens

Questions 379–386

Etta is a 45-year-old G3 P3 who presents at your practice for her annual examination. She is a well-groomed, energetic business woman with 3 children. She works full time and is very active in her community. She initially denies any health problems but then admits to vague abdominal discomfort, similar to feelings of hunger. She also notes occasional epigastric burning 2–3 hours after a meal. These symptoms have been of 2 months' duration. Her vital signs are stable and physical examination is normal. Her abdomen is soft and nontender, and bowel sounds are normal. Her liver, spleen, and kidneys are nonpalpable. A digital rectal exam is negative for masses and hemoccult testing is negative. Her gynecologic examination is within normal limits. Her nutritional history reveals a moderate to low-fat diet. She drinks 3–4 cups of coffee per day, has smoked 5 cigarettes per day for 20 years, and has a glass of wine or alcoholic beverage with dinner 3 times per week. She enjoys dairy products and consumes milk and cheese regularly.

379. What is the most important nonpharmacologic intervention that you could recommend in treating peptic ulcer disease?

(A) Discontinuing alcohol and caffeine intake
(B) Smoking cessation
(C) Frequent feedings of a bland diet

380. What diagnostic test would you order that would be most sensitive in confirming the diagnosis of peptic ulcer disease?

   (A) Endoscopy
   (B) Barium x-ray
   (C) Abdominal ultrasound

381. Etta has a barium x-ray and is found to have evidence of a gastric ulcer. The ulcer measures 2.8×1.5 cm. What would be the next step in her management?

   (A) Begin cimetidine 300 mg po tid and reevaluate in 8 weeks.
   (B) Order endoscopic evaluation and biopsies.
   (C) Counsel the patient on dietary changes that include frequent small meals, bland diet, increased milk consumption, and decreased spices, fruit juices, caffeine, and alcohol.

382. Which risk factor is not associated with peptic ulcer disease?

   (A) Cigarette smoking
   (B) Alcohol use
   (C) First degree relative with ulcer history

383. Many drugs are associated with increasing the risk of peptic ulcer disease. Aspirin is one of these drugs. What statement is true regarding the use of ASA therapy?

   (A) Enteric-coated or buffered aspirin will prevent gastric ulceration.
   (B) The risk of gastric ulcer increases sixfold when patients ingest 1 aspirin tablet daily.
   (C) Aspirin disrupts the gastric mucosa physiologically and anatomically, leading to ulcer formation.

384. What are the causes of duodenal ulcer disease?

   (A) *Helicobacter pylori*
   (B) Chronic stress
   (C) Giardiasis

385. How would one directly identify *H. pylori*?

   (A) Detection of the presence of urease by performing the urea breath test

   (B) Histologic sections abtained at the endoscopic evaluation
   (C) Gastric secretory studies

386. What regimen would you choose in the treatment of duodenal ulcer with evidence of *H. pylori* infection?

   (A) Cimetidine 300 mg po qid
   (B) Omprazole 40–60 mg per day
   (C) Metronidazole 500 mg po tid × 14 days, bismuth 2 tabs po qid × 14 days, tetracycline 500 mg po tid × 14 days

Questions 387–391

Mrs. Yaw, a 50-year-old, overweight mother of 3 teenagers, has a blood pressure (BP) of 120/90 mm Hg on routine screening. Her job and lifestyle are both sedentary. She does not smoke and drinks alcohol "socially." Family history is negative for mother with hypertension.

387. You advise her that

   (A) Her BP is high normal and warrants no further follow-up at this time
   (B) She should have three additional BP checks on three separate occasions
   (C) She is considered to have an established diagnosis of hypertension

388. Repeated exams of Mrs. Yaw by the NP reveal a systolic BP of 120–140 mm Hg and a diastolic of 88–94 mm Hg. The next step in the management of Mrs. Yaw would be to

   (A) Begin a program of nonpharmacologic measures
   (B) Institute a pharmacologic therapy to reduce the patient's short-term risk
   (C) Recheck her BP at her annual visit in 12 months

389. As part of the patient's initial evaluation, you order the following labs to assess target organ damage and Mrs. Yaw's overall cardiac status:

   (A) Echocardiogram to document the presence of left ventricular hypertrophy
   (B) Cardiac lipid profile, complete blood count with differential, fasting blood sugar

(C) Hematocrit, urine analysis, automated blood chemistry, electrocardiogram

390. Mrs. Yaw returns for a blood pressure check in 3 months. Her blood work returned as within normal limits, including her cholesterol profile. However, she had little success with weight loss and was "too busy" to start and maintain an exercise program. Her BP remains consistently in the mild hypertension range. You determine her diagnosis as

(A) Secondary hypertension
(B) Primary hypertension
(C) "White coat" hypertension

391. As first-line therapy, you decide to start the patient on any on the following EXCEPT

(A) Combined alpha/beta blocker
(B) Beta blocker
(C) Angiotensin-converting enzyme (ACE) inhibitor

Questions 392–395

A 52-year-old elementary school bus driver has rectal itching, rectal irritation and rectal discomfort, which is made worse by straining with bowel movements. She has no previous history of bowel dysfunction except constipation. She also experiences occasional bright red rectal staining when constipated. Her history is significant for frequent tension headaches for which she takes ibuprofen as needed. Nonprescription medications include a multivitamin qd and vitamins A, beta carotene and vitamin C in large doses for the "antioxidants" and "free radicals." Physical exam reveals a bluish, firm varix protruding around the superior portion of the anus. There is no excoriation, laceration, fissure, rash, or other lesions. Family history negative for polyps or colon cancer.

392. Your diagnostic impression is

(A) Tinea cruris
(B) Hemorrhoids
(C) Pinworms

393. In order to rule out tinea in this client you would order

(A) Stool for ova and parasites
(B) Potassium hydroxide (KOH)
(C) A series of three to five cellophane tape preparations

394. The initial treatment of external hemorrhoids in this patient would be

(A) Laxatives
(B) Hemorrhoidectomy
(C) High-fiber diet

395. Advising and teaching this client about the American Cancer Society's (ACS) recommendation for early detection of cancer includes all of the following except

(A) Digital rectal exam annually beginning at age 40 and sigmoidoscopy every 3 years beginning at age 50
(B) Fecal occult blood testing (FOBT) beginning at age 50
(C) Colonoscopy beginning at age 50

Questions 396–399

Helen is a young anxious female with a 3-month history of abdominal bloating, intermittent cramping, and frequent loose stools with mucus. Menses are regular, and weight is stable. She reports sleeping well and is not awakened by her symptoms. She denies nausea, vomiting, melena, occult blood, or fever. Her medications include Depo-Provera and acetaminophen 650 mg prn for "tension" headaches. Physical exam including abdominal, rectal, and thyroid are normal. Stool guaiac is negative for occult blood and compete blood count is normal.

396. Your most likely diagnosis is

(A) Irritable bowel syndrome (IBS)
(B) Inflammatory bowel disease (IBD)
(C) Infectious colitis

397. With Helen, it is important to review the dietary history for

(A) Intake of normoflatulogenic foods
(B) Lactose intolerance
(C) Dietary factors do not influence IBS.

398. Helen's medication history, including antibiotic use, must be reviewed to rule out

(A) *Campylobacter jejuni*
(B) *Clostridium difficile*
(C) Salmonella

399. When diarrhea is the predominant symptom, you would order

(A) Stool for ova and parasites and fecal leukocytes
(B) Serum alkaline phosphatase
(C) Serum amylase

Question 400

A 23-year-old patient woke up 2 nights ago with lower abdominal pain rated as a 2 (on a 1–10 scale with 1 being no pain and 10 most severe pain), which she "felt was muscular." Pain is located below umbilicus and radiates to both sides of abdomen, is dull, and is constant. Patient has not eaten today. She denies bladder irritative symptoms, nausea, vomiting, or diarrhea. LMP 20 days ago is reported as normal. Gynecologic history is significant for mild cervical dysplasia 4 years ago and genital warts 18 months ago. Pain is exacerbated by sitting and turning in bed. Last bowel movement was in the morning of the office visit, described as normal by patient but it "hurt to stand up afterward." Patient denies trauma. Physical examination reveals pulse 80 regular, temperature, 98.5°F, BP 130/95. Patient is walking guardedly. Bowel sounds are hypoactive with tenderness at McBurney's point and with rebound and guarding.

400. What is your diagnostic impression?

(A) Acute appendicitis
(B) Acute cholecystitis
(C) Ectopic pregnancy

Questions 401–405

Ella is a 58-year-old G5 P5 who presents with 2 weeks' duration of chest pain. She describes the pain as burning and squeezing; it is steady and ends gradually. She noticed it initially while raking the lawn. The pain is located in the center of her chest and is sometimes associated with tingling down the inside of her arm to her fingers. She has used non-prescription Zantac without improvement of the symptoms. She recently quit smoking and has gained 20 lb. She is not on any regular medication but takes vitamins and calcium citrate 1500 mg daily. Her father died of an acute MI at age 65 years.

401. The Framingham Heart Study, a longitudinal cohort study started in 1948, included women from the outset. What finding is true concerning women and cardiovascular disease?

(A) The case fatality rate for acute MI is higher in men than women.
(B) Women tend to present with angina as their initial manifestation in contrast to men, who present with acute MI
(C) Diabetes, low HDL levels, and hypertriglyceridemia are equally strong risk factors in both men and women.

402. What is the single diagnostic symptom of myocardial ischemia?

(A) The predictable relationship to exertion, emotional stress, or situations that increase oxygen demand
(B) The description of squeezing, chest pain that is substernal and steady and ends gradually
(C) The ability of the patient to "walk through" the pain until it is resolved

403. Ella's physical exam is normal and her heart sounds are normal without evidence of murmur or irregular rate or rhythm. The clinician orders an ECG, which shows evidence of Q wave and ST abnormalities. What would be the next step in her evaluation?

(A) Stress test
(B) Coronary arteriography
(C) Chest x-ray

404. Screening for modifiable risk factors can have a significant impact on a patient's future health. Which is the most significant risk factor for this patient?

(A) Sedentary lifestyle
(B) Smoking status
(C) 20 lb weight gain

405. The clinician orders a diagnostic workup for cardiovascular disease and discusses some options for management. The clinician discusses hormone replacement therapy (HRT) as one option. The PEPI Study found which of the following to be true?

(A) Estrogen and progesterone replacement protect the heart by a 40–50% reduction in the risk of coronary heart disease.
(B) Micronized progesterone had a more favorable impact on HDL when compared to progesterone acetate.
(C) Estrogen and combined estrogen plus progesterone regimens had similar impacts on increasing HDL and decreasing LDL levels.

Questions 406–408

Tina is a 65-year-old healthy woman who complains of severe, persistent back pain that preceded a skin rash located on the left lateral aspect of her trunk. The sharp, tingling pain does not seem to be improving and the rash is spreading over her left side, with the lesions draining a clear fluid. She denies fever and chills but complains of fatigue and insomnia. She noticed the onset of the skin eruptions 2 days ago.

406. The clinician evaluates the lesions, which are a cluster of coalescing vesicles located on the left lateral area of the back. Which test would be appropriate at this point?

(A) Herpes titre
(B) Tzanck smear
(C) Sedimentation rate

407. Which statement is true regarding herpes zoster?

(A) Patients with a history of varicella have a decreased risk of developing herpes zoster.
(B) Patients who are diagnosed with herpes zoster frequently develop a prodrome of pain in the affected dermatome.
(C) Treatment with acyclovir can be initiated any time during the course of disease and significantly decreases the duration of the outbreak.

408. The clinician examines the patient's face for evidence of lesion development. She performs an ophthalmoscopic exam for evidence of eye involvement. Which complication is associated with lesions involving the trigeminal dermatome?

(A) Facial palsy
(B) Deafness
(C) Secondary glaucoma

Questions 409–411

Clarisse is a 67-year-old G5 P5 who has an appointment for her annual examination. The patient admits to being in good health with a history of hypertension treated with Zestril. The clinician questions Clarisse about any changes in her health status and she admits to pain and swelling in her hands. She notes early morning stiffness that resolves after 15 or 20 minutes. She hears cracking when she moves her joints. She denies redness over the joints. She has no fatigue or malaise and continues to volunteer in the local elementary school.

409. The clinician examines the patient's hands and notes bony enlargement of the distal interphalangeal joints. What is this clinical sign called?

(A) Heberden's nodes
(B) Raynaud's Phenomenon
(C) Subchondral cysts

410. What clinical findings are *not* commonly associated with early onset of osteoarthritis?

(A) Absence of systemic clinical symptoms
(B) Bony enlargement and irregularity of the joint
(C) Heat and redness over the joint

411. The clinician orders blood work and an x-ray of the patient's hands. What findings will point to a diagnosis of osteoarthritis?

(A) Rheumatoid factor 1:80
(B) Elevated C-reactive protein
(C) Abnormal x-ray findings

Questions 412–414

An elderly woman presents with a 2-day history of facial pain. She has had cold symptoms for approximately 3 weeks. She also complains of nasal stuffiness and yellowish green nasal discharge. She is allergic to dust, pollen, and molds. Smoking history is negative with no significant exposure to passive smoke. Physical exam reveals frontal and maxillary sinus tenderness, erythematous nasal mucosa with boggy turbinates, no fever, and a normal neurologic exam. The pharynx is unremarkable and there is no cervical adenopathy. Ear exam is negative.

412.   The most likely diagnosis is

(A) Temporomandibular joint (TMJ) pain

(B) Acute sinusitis

(C) Migraine headache

413.   Your next step in the management of this patient would be to

(A) Treat with rest, fluids, and hydration

(B) Order sinus films

(C) Treat with an appropriate antibiotic and monitor response to therapy

414.   The drug of choice to treat the organism implicated in sinusitis (*S. pneumoniae* [31–36%], *H. influenza* [21–23%], *Moraxella catarrhalis* [2–19%]) would be

(A) Amoxicillin 500 mg po bid × 14 days

(B) Erythromycin 250 mg po qid × 10 days

(C) Tetracycline 500 mg po qid × 7 days

Answers and Rationales
for Primary Care Cases

302. **(A)** The second intercostal space or aortic area is where S_1 is softer than S_2. Also S_1 is softer than S_2 at the second left intercostal space or number 2 on the picture of the chest wall. The S_1 sound is mitral valve and tricuspid valve closure and so would be softer at the base of the heart.

303. **(C)** The apex of the heart is where S_1 is usually louder than S_2. At the position labeled 4, splitting of the second heart sound may be heard. The S_2 sound is aortic and pulmonic closure and so would be softer at the apex of the heart.

304. **(C)** The mitral valve sounds are best heard at the apex of the heart. If you ask the client to roll onto the left side and place the bell on the apical impulse, this will help assess for mitral murmurs.

305. **(B)** Aortic murmurs are accentuated by asking the client to sit up, lean forward, exhale completely, and stop breathing in expiration and then listening with the diaphragm of the stethoscope at the left sternal border.

306. **(B)** Smoking typically begins in the teen years or early adulthood. In the past, males were more likely to smoke than females. But this is no longer the case. Social influences such as peer pressure are major factors in initiating smoking. There is no "smoker" personality type, though smokers tend to be more adventuresome/risk taking and extroverted. Cigarette smoking runs in families and is thought to be due to a social modeling process.

307. **(A)** Primary prevention needs to be directed at adolescents and preadolescents. Ideally, formal preventive intervention begins between fourth and sixth grade. Education needs to include specific instructions and role-playing about resisting offers to use cigarettes, alcohol, and illicit drugs. Adolescents exposed to "resistance training" either are less likely to smoke or initiate smoking at later ages. Discussing the negative effect of smoking and the benefits of quitting at each visit is also helpful.

Only a small number of patients attend smoking-cessation support groups when they are available for little or no cost. Smoking-cessation support groups have had limited success. Fear is a weak motivator in changing complex behaviors.

308. **(B)** Since carbon monoxide and nicotine are mainly responsible for cardiovascular disease and cleared within hours of smoking cessation, there is a reduction in cardiac work requirement and an increase in oxygenation. There is also a reduction in upper respiratory infection. Benefits in cancer reduction risk and pulmonary status are measurable within 3–5 years of smoking cessation. Weight gain of 5–15 lb the first year is considered of *no* major consequence relative to the benefits of smoking cessation.

309. **(C)** Lung function will be generally normal unless respiratory illness is present.

310. **(B)** Due to the increase in smoking by women, lung cancer mortality has risen steadily since the mid-1960s; lung cancer is now the leading cause of cancer deaths in women.

311. **(A)** She is at risk for future problems due to frequent binge drinking. Binge drinking is

especially prevalent among adolescents. Most frequent binge drinkers have numerous alcohol-related problems, including problems with school work, unplanned or unsafe sex, and trouble with police.

312. **(A)** Heavy drinkers may underestimate the amount they drink because of denial, forgetfulness, or fear of the consequences of being diagnosed with a drinking problem.

313. **(A)** The four-question CAGE instrument is the most popular screening test for use in primary care, though it may be less specific in young persons. The CAGE may be less sensitive for early problem drinking and hazardous drinking. The four-question CAGE instrument is as follows:

    C: "Have you ever felt you ought to **C**ut down on drinking?"
    A: "Have people **A**nnoyed you by criticizing you drinking?"
    For use in primary care:
    G: "Have you ever felt bad or **G**uilty about your drinking?"
    E: "Have you ever had a drink first thing in the morning to steady your nerves or get rid of a hangover (**E**ye opener)?"

    The MAST is too lengthy for routine screening. The AUDIT, developed by the World Health Organization (WHO), is a 10-item screening instrument that may detect a broader range of current drinking problems but its use in primary care needs further evaluation. Alternative drinking screens are being devised for adolescents.

314. **(C)** Of migraine sufferers, 20–50% have a positive family history, usually in one parent. Onset of migraines is usually between ages 15 and 25; they are more common in women. An initial stage of vasoconstriction, producing brain ischemia, results in various symptoms, including aura. Prodromal warning helps establish the diagnosis. Unilateral pain that reaches a peak in several hours to a day is typical. The pain is pounding or throbbing. Recurrence is a hallmark of migraine. Most migraine sufferers have several attacks each year. Migraines become less frequent and less severe with age.

315. **(B)** Frequent symptoms accompanying migraine headaches are nausea, vomiting, and intolerance to light (photophobia) and sound. Perimenstrual period (before the onset of bleeding when estradiol levels are falling), oral contraceptives (especially off days, presumably due to falling estrogen levels), and menopause are associated with migraine episodes. The following substances may initiate migraines in susceptible women: vasodilators (nitrates and antihypertensives); alcohol; chocolate; cheese, wines, and other foods containing tryamine; and monosodium glutamate.

316. **(B)** Ergotamine is the treatment of choice at the onset of prodromal symptoms. It has a short shelf life and should not be used more than twice in the same week. Because of its specificity, ergotamine can be used at therapeutic trial to establish the diagnosis. For mild attacks, acetaminophen, aspirin, or another antiinflammatory used in the treatment of tension headaches give relief. Avoiding triggers and reclining in a cool dark room are helpful measures. Prophylactic therapies used most are propranolol, amitriptyline, and calcium channel blockers.

317. **(C)** Tension (muscle contraction) headache symptoms are presumed to be caused by contractions of scalp and neck muscles. Pain is usually bilateral, and recurs with similar quality and location. A history of psychosocial stress is often associated with headache episodes. Patients may get some relief with scalp massage. Physical exam is unremarkable except for neck or scalp muscle tenderness. In the differential diagnosis of headache, one of the most important considerations is TIAs, especially in middle-age and older patients. Cluster headaches occur predominantly in middle-aged men who are thin and smoke.

318. **(A)** Accutane (isotretinoin) is curative in many patients with cystic acne, although the exact mechanism is unknown. The greatest concern is the teratogenic potential. This drug may produce fetal anomalies involving the central nervous system, heart, bones, and thy-

mus in 30–40% of exposed fetuses. Sexually active patients should be counseled in choosing a very reliable contraceptive. If pregnancy occurs, the option of abortion should be discussed. Patient instructions and drug consent forms are available from the manufacturer.

319. **(B)** Mild elevations of triglyceride, cholesterol, and liver enzymes commonly occur. Patients are usually treated with Accutane for approximately 20 weeks. Triglycerides, cholesterol, and liver enzymes should be checked prior to treatment and at monthly intervals. If triglyceride levels double or triple, appropriate diet modifications and avoidance of alcohol should be instituted. If levels exceed 500, Accutane should be stopped or reduced in dose with testing every 1–2 weeks. Minor elevations in liver enzymes require no treatment. If two- to threefold elevations occur, other causes of aminotransferase elevations should be explored. The patient should be cautioned to avoid alcohol. Patients on Accutane should be seen monthly to evaluate clinical improvement, to review contraceptive behavior, and to perform lab tests. Pregnancy testing at each visit is strongly recommended.

320. **(A)** Common side effects of Accutane therapy include xerosis (dry skin) and xerophthalmia (dry eyes). Infrequent side effects are hair loss, musculoskeletal aches, *Staphylococcus aureus* folliculitis and ocular keratitis, reduced night vision, and markedly elevated lipids and liver enzymes.

321. **(A)** The status of a woman's health can influence not only her ability to conceive but also her ability to maintain the pregnancy. The National Institute of Health and Human Services expert panel reviewed the factors that contribute to favorable pregnancy outcomes for women and infants and recommended prenatal care begin prior to conception, preferably within 1 year of a planned pregnancy.

Areas to focus on are menstrual cycles (advise patient to keep a record), exercise and nutrition, teratogen avoidance, identification of unhealthy behaviors, identification and appropriate referral of medical conditions, identification of genetic risk with pedigree, immunizations, psychosocial and financial issues, lab tests (hematocrit and hemoglobin, Rh, GC, VDRL, chlamydia, Pap, urine for protein, sugar, leukocytes, TB, and HIV if risk factors).

322. **(B)** Organogenesis occurs between day 17 and day 56 after fertilization. Thus many compromised pregnancy outcomes are determined before women have had an opportunity to begin care.

323. **(B)** Prior to conception, prospective parents can make informed lifestyle decisions to maximize the chance of a healthy pregnancy outcome. Preconception counseling should take place routinely during physical exams when women are contemplating pregnancy. Actual and potential risk factors need to be assessed.

324. **(A)** In 1992 the U.S. Public Health Service Center for Disease Control announced new recommendations in the periconception period. Women with a history of an affected pregnancy are at particular risk in subsequent pregnancies. Food sources rich in folate are leafy, dark-green vegetables; citrus fruits and juices; yeast; bread; beans; and fortified breakfast cereals. The preconception visit offers an opportunity to counsel about the needs for increased protein, calcium, and calories and to prepare women for the weight gain and body-image changes that accompany pregnancy.

325. **(A)** The typical case of rheumatoid arthritis (RA) begins with slow progression of symptoms and signs over a period of months to weeks. Arthritic symptoms include stiffness in one or more joints accompanied by pain and tenderness with movement. The patient is able to bear weight but notes persistent, deep, gnawing discomfort. Fatigue, malaise, and depression may precede other symptoms of the disease. The patient denies fatigue upon waking but notices it 4–6 hours later. The number of joints involved usually progresses to involve five or more and is sequential in its pattern of involvement, ie, from fingers to hands to wrists to elbows. The axial skeletal is often spared.

326. (B) Pregnancy is often responsible for a remission of rheumatoid arthritis symptoms. Recurrence of pain and swelling recur about 6 weeks postpartum.

327. (B) The usual starting dose of aspirin therapy is 900 mg 4 times per day. The drug should be enteric coated to minimize gastric upset. There is a narrow margin between therapeutic and toxic levels of aspirin. The earliest symptom of toxicity is tinnitus or mild deafness. Aspirin should be discontinued until the symptoms resolve and then restarted at a lower dose.

328. (C) Rheumatoid antibodies are detectable in 70–80% of patients with the disease. A significant titre is 1:80 or greater. RF usually becomes positive within 6 months of the onset of disease. Rheumatoid factor is also detectable in the normal population, more commonly in persons greater than 50 years of age. RF is also positive in patients presumed to have chronic antigenic stimulation such as in prolonged infectious states, ie, bacterial endocarditis, tuberculosis, viral hepatitis, and chronic lung disease. Recent vaccination may cause a transient rise in rheumatoid factor.

329. (B) The American Rheumatism Association includes the following criteria needed to diagnose rheumatoid arthritis: (1) persistent swelling of the joints for longer than 6 weeks' duration; (2) soft tissue swelling (or increased fluid) in a joint followed by swelling of symmetrical joints.

330. (B) The criteria for diagnosis of major clinical depression is a depressed mood for at least a 2-week period as well as five of the following symptoms: weight loss or weight gain, insomnia or hypersomnia, psychomotor agitation or retardation, fatigue or loss of energy, feelings of worthlessness or excessive guilt, diminished ability to think, and recurrent thoughts of death and/or suicide. PMS is related to menstrual cycle and is prior to menses. Thyroid problems may cause weight changes and mood swings but the best choice is depression.

331. (C) Marital status is not a risk factor for depression. Women are more likely than men to develop depression. Depression occurs 6–12% in women and 2–5% in men. A major life stress event frequently is involved with onset of symptoms. Depression is more common in families with a history of a relative with depression. The cause may be related to learned coping patterns or a biological component. It is not clearly understood. Both married and single women are at risk. A woman with a history of depression in the past is at risk for postpartum depression.

332. (A) Prozac is classified as a category B drug in pregnancy. It does not cause orthostatic hypotension, constipation, or sedation. In a recent study comparing first-trimester treatment with Prozac, standard tricyclics, and no treatment, there were no differences regarding miscarriages and congenital abnormalities. Also, there is a Prozac pregnancy registry that has followed over 1000 births with no reported fetal abnormalities. It is important to weigh the risks and benefits with the client and decide about treatment options.

333. (A) Maternity blues, baby blues, or postpartum blues is experienced by approximately 50% of women within 3–6 days after delivery. Symptoms include insomnia, weepiness, anxiety, irritability, and poor concentration. The symptoms are mild and last only a few hours as opposed to more than 2 weeks, as in postpartum depression. Postpartum depression begins 3–6 months after delivery and follows the criteria for major clinical depression listed in answer 330 above, in which you need to have 5 of the symptoms with a depressed mood for the diagnosis. Women with a prior history of postpartum depression have a 70% chance of a recurrence.

334. (A) Oral contraceptives may increase the effects of corticosteroids by decreasing their clearance and increasing their half-life. Thus this client may need a lower steroid dose. OCs may decrease the clearance of benzodiazepines such as diazepam, chlordiazepoxide, and alprazolam.

335. **(B)** Oral contraceptives can alter thyroid function by elevating thyroid-binding globulin and decreasing free thyroxin.

336. **(B)** High doses of vitamin C (ascorbic acid) increase the serum level of ethinyl estradiol by 50% in OC users. Thus, a low-dose pill is in effect changed to a high-dose pill. Intermittent use of high doses of vitamin C can cause spotting when the vitamin is discontinued. If she insists on taking a vitamin C supplement, she should take it at a different time than her birth control pills—at least 4 hours apart. Taking 1 g of vitamin C daily to boost the immune system and prevent colds is not recommended for women on OCs.

337. **(B)** Women on anticonvulsants such as phenobarbital, phenytoin, carbamazepine, primidone, and ethosuximides (the anticonvulsant sodium valproate does not have this effect) should be started on a higher dose OC containing 50 μg of ethinyl estradiol *Note*: Rifampin also has potent enzyme-inducing effects, as does the antifungal drug griseofulvin.

338. **(B)** There is no firm pharmacokinetic evidence that links antibiotic use to altered steroid blood levels. There are only anecdotal case reports of contraceptive failure in OC users on antibiotics.

339. **(B)** Patients with basal cell nevus syndrome, with xeroderma or multiple nonmelanoma skin cancers may be treated with retinoids. At appropriate doses of isotretinoin or etretinate, patients have lower rates of recurrence. The retinoid must be continued indefinitely to maintain the protective effect. Potential side effects of retinoid use include lipid elevations, calcification of tendons, and hyperostosis.

340. **(B)** The lesion should be biopsied to confirm the diagnosis prior to treatment. Treatment modality depends on the type of cancer. Most often lesions are removed with excisional biopsy.

341. **(A)** The major risk factors for nonmelanoma skin cancers are cumulative sun exposure, skin color, and age. Individuals with fair skin and inability to tan are at increased risk for skin damage. Most nonmelanoma skin cancers occur on sun-exposed surfaces but may occur on covered sites such as the scalp or genitalia. Patients who have undergone organ transplants and immunosuppressive therapy have a 4–21-fold increase in risk of skin cancer 10 years after organ transplant. Certain disorders such as basal cell nevus syndrome and xeroderma pigmentosum increase the early onset of skin cancer.

342. **(C)** Hepatitis B vaccine is a recombinant vaccine made in yeast and may be given to this patient. Patients with a history of allergic reaction associated with eating eggs should not receive yellow fever and influenza vaccines, which are made in eggs.

343. **(B)** Passive immunization with immune globulin is 90% effective in preventing hepatitis A in exposed individuals. IG should be offered to family and intimate contacts. IG should be given as soon as possible following exposure. Hepatitis A vaccines are available in Europe and the United States but are given for preventive cases in high-risk situations.

344. **(B)** Tetanus commonly occurs following animal bites and penetrating wounds. The majority of cases occur in persons over 60 years of age who were never immunized. The primary series consists of three doses in childhood with a booster of absorbed toxoid every 10 years. Boosters may be needed for serious wounds if the patient has not had a booster within 5 years. Summary guides to tetanus prophylaxis are available from the CDC.

345. **(B)** Influenza vaccine works optimally in healthy young adults and exhibits lower rates of effectiveness in elderly and debilitated persons. The vaccine is most effective when close matches of *antigens* from predicted strains and viruses are made for the future flu season.

346. **(C)** Arthralgias will be experienced by up to 40% of adults within 1–3 weeks following immunization with rubella. Most symptoms are mild and transient. The measles component of MMR is responsible for the fever and rash 5–12 days following injection.

347. **(B)** The majority of cases of hepatitis are anicteric. Patients have few nonspecific symptoms such as fatigue and nausea and the disease is often misdiagnosed as a flu-like illness. The correct diagnosis is made by demonstrating bilirubin in the urine.

348. **(A)** Type A hepatitis, previously known as infectious hepatitis, is the most common type. It is primarily transmitted by the oral–fecal route. Poor hygienic conditions where people are in close contact increase the spread of the virus. Fecal contamination of water or food supplies and ingestion of shellfish contribute to outbreaks.

349. **(C)** The patient usually seeks medical attention with the appearance of dark urine, pruritus, and jaundice. A tender, palpable liver may be found on physical exam in 70% of patients. Posterior cervical lymphadenopathy and splenomegaly may also be present. Jaundice peaks within a few days and resolves completely by 2–8 weeks from onset of disease.

350. **(B)** The serum aminotransferases rise before the onset of jaundice and may elevate to several thousand units and remain abnormal for several weeks. The persistent elevation is of no prognostic value. However, the serum total bilirubin rise is an indication of severity of disease.

351. **(C)** A rapid fall in serum aminotransferases from a high peak value to normal in less than 1 week may be an indication of fulminant hepatitis with a collapse of liver parenchyma. A prolonged prothrombin time with no response to vitamin K therapy is suggestive of severe hepatitis. If the prothrombin time is further prolonged, it indicates fulminant hepatitis. Fulminant hepatitis is more commonly associated with type B and is the principal cause of death in hepatitis patients. This occurs more commonly in debilitated patients and those patients with coexisting disease.

352. **(B)** Most patients clear hepatitis B surface antigen within 3 months of the onset of illness. When patients have clinical or laboratory evidence of liver disease, chronic hepatitis and cirrhosis should be suspected and the patient referred to a liver specialist. The incidence of progressive liver disease is 3–5% with type B and 20–50% in type C hepatitis. Liver biopsy is indicated when disease extends beyond 6 months.

353. **(A)** Patients with alcoholic hepatitis present with fever and leukocytosis. A liver biopsy should be taken to differentiate alcoholic, drug-induced, and viral hepatitis. Alcoholic hepatitis is often more severe and one third of patients may progress to liver cirrhosis. Abstinence from drinking alcohol increases chances of complete recovery. Women are more susceptible to alcohol-induced hepatitis and the disease is dose dependent. Women can develop liver damage after consuming less than 20 g per day whereas men usually consume at least 60 g per day before onset of disease (½ oz straight alcohol = 15g).

354. **(A)** Elevations of serum aminotransferases and alkaline phosphatase are occasionally found in healthy subjects or those without liver disease. Repeat testing should confirm the elevation. Elevated serum aminotransferases can originate from injury to the heart or striated muscle. A recent bone fracture can result in an elevated serum alkaline phosphatase. If muscle injury is sustained, the creatine kinase will be elevated. The hepatic origin of elevated alkaline phosphatese can be confirmed by an elevated 5'-nucleotidase, which is present only in the liver and bile ducts.

355. **(B)** Flexible or rigid sigmoidoscopy is usually the first test done in the evaluation of the lower bowel. The finding of hemorrhoids, polyps, or even rectal cancer does not negate the need to evaluate the rest of the colon. If the results are inconclusive, barium enema or colonoscopy should be performed. Patients under 40 years of age with bleeding patterns consistent with rectal disease and absence of a rectal lesion on proctosigmoidoscopy may

need surveillance with rectal examination and hemoccult testing.

356. **(C)** Smoking is not a risk factor for colon cancer until the patient has smoked greater than 35 years. Studies have shown that cigarette smoking may decrease the risk of colon cancer in the early years of use. In one study, smokers of 35 years' duration or greater had a high relative risk of cancer, which increased the longer the woman continued to smoke (Sandler, 1988).

357. **(B)** False-negative results are caused by ingesting high doses of vitamin C. False-positive results may be increased by laxative use, peroxidase-rich foods (red meat, broccoli, turnips, and cauliflower), and iron compounds. Laxative use increases the number of true positives and true negatives of the hemoccult test possibly by causing an irritative effect on the colon.

358. **(A)** It is believed that all colon cancers excluding those associated with ulcerative colitis have originated from a benign epithelial tumor. It is estimated that it takes at least 5 years for a polyp to grow into an invasive cancer. Early detection and removal of the benign lesion is significant. The risk of polyps becoming malignant is related to the histologic type and size. Hyperplastic polyps have very little malignant potential. Villous and tubular adenomas carry a definite risk of cancer.

359. **(A)** The individual with familial atypical mole and melanoma syndrome (FAMM) begins to develop atypical lesions at puberty and continues to develop new lesions throughout life. The three criteria describing this syndrome are: family history of melanoma in at least one first- or second-degree relative, the presence of many nevi, and atypical histologic patterns. Persons with FAMM have a lifetime risk of developing melanoma that approaches 100%.

360. **(A)** A typical mole or nevus is round, is brown to tan in color, and has well demarcated borders. Most benign lesions are present since early adulthood and the average adult has 20 typical nevi. Dysplastic nevi are larger than usual moles, are irregular in shape, and have poorly defined borders. Pigmentation is variable and may include black, brown, blue, red, and/or tan coloration.

361. **(B)** The patient should be counseled to avoid prolonged exposure to direct sunlight, which increases the risk of malignancy. She should apply sun screen to all exposed skin surfaces on a daily basis. She should understand that sunscreen is not protective when it is used to enable the patient to be exposed to several hours of direct sunlight. Monthly self-examination of skin and clinical examinations every 4–6 months are advised. Photographs and skin mapping can be used to follow lesion progression and to identify new lesions.

362. **(C)** The thyroid hormones in the blood are T_4 and a smaller quantity of T_3. The majority of the plasma thyroid hormones are bound to several plasma proteins but a small percentage is freely circulating in the plasma and reflects the amount of hormone exerting an effect on the tissue. The most important measurements of thyroid function are of the levels of T_4 and T_3 as determined by radioimmunoassay. The value of T_4 is considered the single most important measurement of thyroid disease but must be interpreted as accurate only if the T_4 binding to plasma proteins is normal. In practice this is done by measuring the free T_4 index. Although the T_4 is the most valuable level, the appropriate lab test for measurement is the free T_4. The TSH is the most sensitive test for diagnosis of hypothyroidism.

363. **(C)** Chronic liver disease produces many abnormalities in an unpredictable fashion. T_4 may be increased or decreased in parallel with thyroid binding globulin. T_3 is often decreased. The TSH value is frequently elevated. Thyroid binding globulin and T_4 are both elevated during pregnancy and estrogen therapy.

364. **(B)** Increased vascularity of the gland may result in palpable or audible blood flow over the thyroid gland. A bruit is usually heard

over the enlarged lobes or over the superior thyroid arteries. A bruit heard over the thyroid of a hyperthyroid patient is diagnostic of Graves' disease as it is not present in patients with toxic nodular goiter.

365. **(C)** Clinical symptoms and signs of hyperthyroidism include tremulousness, anxiety, weight loss, sweats, and heat intolerance. Palpitations may also occur. Physical findings include tachycardia, thyroid enlargement, and a fine tremor. Laboratory values will be an elevated T_4, T_3, and FTI. TSH will be decreased.

366. **(C)** An optimal choice would be to abruptly stop the medications and recheck the freeT_4 and TSH in 5 weeks. If the patient has a true diagnosis, her symptoms will be diagnostic of the thyroid disease.

367. **(B)** Although laboratory evidence of a euthyroid state may exist, it takes several months for the normal metabolic state to be restored. A change in the laboratory value of T_4 takes approximately 6–8 weeks. The objective of therapy is to maintain the plasma T_4 at the mid to upper range of normal. When the T_4 reaches the normal range, the TSH can be performed for fine tuning. The value of the TSH should also be within the normal range.

368. **(B)** T_4 is the choice of hormones tested in titrating thyroid replacement therapy. TSH should be tested when the T_4 reaches the middle to upper range of normal. The T_3 is not considered the test of choice in evaluating hormone replacement. However, in cases of hyperthyroidism where the T_4 is normal, a T_3 should always be evaluated because T_3 is the predominant hormone secreted in 5% of hyperthyroidism associated with Graves' disease, multinodular goiter, and autonomous adenoma.

369. **(B)** The correct interval between initiating therapy or adjusting the dosage and testing serum levels is 6–8 weeks.

370. **(B)** The standard interval is annually unless the patient reports any adverse symptoms.

The patient should be instructed in the use, side effects, and risks of her medication. She should also be educated to recognize symptoms of hypo- and hyperthyroid states.

371. **(A)** Low-pitched voice changes are associated with hypothyroidism. Abnormal eye findings are associated with increased sympathetic tone and the hyperthyroid state. Hand tremors are a common finding in hyperthyroid disease.

372. **(B)** The needle biopsy for cytologic examination is considered the procedure of choice. A scintiscan uses a radioisotope as contrast material to identify whether a nodule is hot or cold. A hot nodule is considered to be benign 99.8% of the time and a cold nodule benign 75–95% of the time. This test is not diagnostic and further workup is necessary. Excision of the thyroid nodule for diagnostic purposes is not the standard of practice in the medical community at the present time, although a complete histologic sample would definitively rule out malignancy.

373. **(B)** Cold nodules are benign 75–95% of the time compared to the hot nodule, which is benign 98% of the time. Single nodules are more likely to be malignant than a multinodular goiter.

374. **(B)** Anaplastic carcinoma is uncommon and highly aggressive and invasive. The cancer quickly produces pain, hoarseness, dysphagia, and hemoptysis. Death occurs within 6–12 months. Medullary carcinoma accounts for 1–2% of thyroid cancers with excellent prognosis following surgical excision with negative nodes. Follicular cancer may metastasize to bones and lungs, bypassing the lymph nodes.

375. **(B)** Current research shows that lesbians often delay seeking treatment and utilize health care services mainly for crisis intervention. General health care screening and ongoing risk assessment and preventive care throughout the life cycle are an integral part of care for all women. Most lesbians feel that their health care will be

positively influenced by revealing their sexual orientation but encountering negative reactions may prevent such disclosure and subsequent seeking of routine health care visits.

376. **(B)** Gonorrhea, chlamydia, and syphilis are rare among lesbians who are sexually active with women only. Clinicians must not assume low risk without exploring past history of sexual exposure since 75–80% of lesbians have had heterosexual experiences. Genital infections with herpes simplex virus and human papilloma virus have been reported in lesbian populations. Cervical dysplasia has also been documented and is a concern as lesbians often delay annual Pap smear screening.

377. **(C)** Studies that address cancer risks specific to lesbians are not available. Currently, prospective studies that stratify women according to sexual preference and experience are ongoing and will attempt to identify risks for specific populations. Breast cancer risks that may impact lesbians disproportionately may include nulliparity, older age at first pregnancy, and absence of lactation experience. Other factors that may reflect decreased access to routine health care are infrequent mammography and breast examination.

378. **(C)** Lesbian teenagers have an increased risk of homelessness, suicide or attempted suicide, and substance abuse. Adolescents with confusion about sexual orientation may present with depression, substance abuse, poor academic performance, and suicidal ideation or attempts. Lesbian teens are 2–3 times more likely to attempt suicide compared to heterosexual teens. A nonjudgmental, supportive provider may be an excellent source of validation and information for youths and teenagers who identify as lesbian.

379. **(B)** The most important nonpharmacologic intervention is smoking cessation. Cigarette smoking increases the risk of PUD and delays healing of the ulcer. Alcohol and caffeine increase acid secretion but discontinuing these substances is not associated with an increase in resolution of the disease. Dietary modifica-

tion does not seem to affect the course of peptic ulcer disease. Bland diet and decreased consumption of spices or fruit juices do not have an impact on healing.

380. **(A)** An experienced endoscopist will diagnose 85–95% of gastroduodenal ulcers. The sensitivity of radiography increases when using both ulcers and erosions as diagnostic criteria. The success in detecting both duodenal and gastric lesions with radiography is 54% compared to 90% for endoscopy.

381. **(B)** The American Society of Gastrointestinal Endoscopy recommends that all patients with gastric ulcers that appear benign with radiologic studies have endoscopy with biopsies at some point in therapy and 8 weeks post initiation of therapy. This is the recommendation for ulcers that are less than 2.5 cm size. The recommendation of early endoscopy following radiologic studies is advised in all patients with ulcers that are not clearly benign or that are greater that 2.5 cm in size. The argument for endoscopic examination in all patients is that 3–7% of benign-appearing lesions will be malignant but appear to be healed on follow-up X-ray studies. There is no evidence that dietary modification affects the course of peptic ulcer disease.

382. **(B)** Alcohol is known to cause acute gastritis but is not thought to be ulcerogenic. Cigarette smoking is associated with increased frequency in this disease. Genetic factors appear to play a role. Duodenal ulcer is three times as common in first-degree relatives.

383. **(C)** In experimental studies aspirin disrupts the gastric mucosa both physiologically and autonomically, leading to ulcer formation. Aspirin use also increases the risk of bleeding from peptic ulcers. The patient must ingest 3 aspirin per day to increase her risk sixfold. Enteric and buffered aspirin have no advantage over regular aspirin with respect to increased risk of ulcer formation.

384. **(A)** *Helicobacter pylori* is a gram-negative spiral organism exclusive to the gastric

epithelium. The organism is prevalent in 10% of healthy people under age 30 years and in 60% of healthy people over age 60 years. The organism is probably spread via direct contact and the rate of infection is more prevalent in lower socioeconomic groups. *H. pylori* is present in the stomach of more than 90% of patients with duodenal ulcer. Eradication of the organism appears to result in accelerated duodenal ulcer healing and decreased recurrence at 1 and 2 years following treatment.

385.   **(B)** Biopsies obtained at the endoscopic evaluation are the most direct way of identifying the presence of the organism. *H. pylori* can also be cultured from the gastric mucosa to get direct results. *H. pylori* can be detected by tests that measure the level of urease by a breath urea test. This seems to be a sensitive but indirect indicator of the presence of *H. pylori*.

386.   **(C)** Triple-therapy regimens are the most common today with very high cure rates and less recurrence at the follow-up visit. Smokers and patients with a coexistent gastric ulcer are less likely to commit to therapy.

387.   **(B)** The diagnosis of hypertension should be made only after elevation is noted on three readings on different occasions with intervals of 2 weeks or more between sets. The patient should have rested ≥ 10 minutes and be in warm surroundings. During a 24-hour ambulatory monitoring, pressures may vary more than 30 mm Hg, with highest levels usually noted in the early morning and lower readings in the afternoon. The average of multiple readings taken over 1–2 months should be taken to establish the diagnosis and decide upon the need for therapy.

Diastolic blood pressure (DBP) between 85 and 89 mm Hg is classified as "high normal," indicating added risk for these patients. DBP 90–104 is considered mild hypertension; DBP 105–114, moderate hypertension; DBP 115 and above, severe hypertension. Systolic (with DBP < 90) 140–159 is borderline isolated systolic hypertension; 160 and above, isolated systolic hypertension.

388.   **(A)** Weight loss (to within 15% of ideal body weight), reducing dietary fat and cholesterol, salt restriction, limiting alcohol intake to no more than 1 oz per day, exercising 20–30 minutes at least three times per week at 80% maxium heart rate, maintaining an adequate intake of potassium, calcium, and magnesium, and using a form of relaxation therapy are the mainstays of nonpharmacologic therapies. This patient does not smoke, but stopping smoking has a major effect in improving overall cardiovascular health.

Patients with uncomplicated mild hypertension (defined as DBP between 90 and 104 mm Hg) need not be started immediately on antihypertensive drugs. Patients are at little short-term risk and will not be endangered by postponement of drug therapy until the permanence of hypertension is determined and nondrug therapies are given a chance to lower the DBP below 90 mm Hg.

389.   **(C)** Hypertension is not just one problem with excessive pressure within the vessels, but a syndrome of multiple abnormalities including insulin resistance and glucose intolerance, hyperlipidemia, and a tendency to develop left ventricular hypertrophy. Lab workup would incude hematocrit (to detect anemia), complete urinalysis (to detect hematuria, proteinuria, and casts, which may signal primary renal disease) and automated blood chemistry, including creatinine (to assess renal parenchymal disease), fasting glucose (to detect diabetes), sodium, potassium (to detect hyperaldosteronism), and total cholesterol and HDL cholesterol (to indicate atherosclerosis risk). An electrocardiogram should also be obtained though echocardiogram is considered more a sensitive indice of left ventricular hypertrophy much earlier than electrocardiography.

390.   **(B)** Primary hypertension or essential hypertension is elevated blood pressure with no specific cause that can be identified. In the typical primary care practice, 95% of hypertensive adults age 18–65 have no identifiable cause. It is also termed *idiopathic*.

Secondary hypertension may result from renal parenchymal disease, renal vascular hypertension, coarctation of the aorta, thyroid disease, adrenal hyperfunction (pheochromocytoma, Cushing syndrome, primary aldosteronism), and medicines such as oral contraceptives, glucocorticoids, steroids, and decongestants. Suspect secondary causes if the patient uses birth control pills or steroids, has paroxysms of headache, flushing, palpitations, tachycardia, an abdominal bruit, BP in legs 10 mm Hg lower than in arms, or delayed femoral pulses.

391. **(A)** Four classes of drugs may be choices for initial therapy: diuretics, beta-blockers, ACE inhibitors, and calcium entry channel blockers. Individualized therapy may be recommended on the basis of the special considerations of demographics, lifestyle, concomitant disease, and cost. Combined alpha/beta blockers are considered second-line agents for the treatment of hypertension. The most common side effects from antihypertensive medications are sexual dysfunction, depression, fatigue, and cognitive impairment.

392. **(B)** Straining at stool, constipation, prolonged sitting, and anal infections are contributing factors to hemorrhoids. With external hemorrhoids patients may feel an external mass. When thrombosed, the mass becomes large and very painful, especially during defecation.

393. **(B)** Potassium hydroxide (KOH) allows for visualization of the yeast spores and the diagnosis of tinea. The cellophane tape preparation can be placed against the anus by the patient upon arising, before a bowel movement, and before the perianal area is cleansed. The tape can be examined microscopically under low power (10×) for the pinworm ova (swabs are also commercially available: Pinworm Diagnostic Tapes, Parke-Davis). For a history suggestive of bacterial or parasitic infection, obtain stool culture, stool for ova and parasites, and stool exam for leukocytes.

394. **(C)** Treatment of choice is a high-fiber diet. Psyllium products can be used to increase fiber. Conservative treatment with high-roughage diet and the addition of a bulk-form-

ing agent with psyllium such as Citrucel®, Hydrocil®, Konsyl®, or Metamucil® is recommended. Hemorrhoidectomy surgery is reserved for severe symptoms or complications. Injection therapy is effective, but the recurrence rate is 50%. Laxatives should be avoided as they do not allow smooth bowel evacuations.

395. **(C)** Colonoscopy is advocated for high-risk groups (eg., familial polyposis, ulcerative colitis, cancer family syndrome) and those with abnormal results of FOBT. Referral to a specialist in these high-risk patients is appropriate. Fecal occult blood testing has a high false-positive rate. Reasons for false positive include ingesting peroxidases and gastric irritants such as salicylates and other antiinflammatory agents. Hemorrhoids, diverticulosis, and peptic ulcers can also cause gastrointestinal bleeding. Ascorbic acid and other antioxidants can interfere with the test reagents and give a false positive. Digital rectal exam is recommended, but is of limited value as a screening test for colorectal cancer, as fewer than 10% of colorectal cancers can be palpated by the examining finger. The exam finger is 7–8 cm long, which limits access to the rectal mucosa, which is 11 cm long.

396. **(A)** IBS is classically characterized by alternating diarrhea and constipation, although a subset of patients present mainly with loose frequent stool (up to 4–6 movements per day). If the symptoms have been present for at least 3 months, establish the Manning criteria for diagnosis (abdominal distention, pain relief with bowel action, more frequent stools with the onset of pain, looser stools with the onset of pain, passage of mucus, and the sensation of incomplete evacuation). IBS may be associated with varying degrees of anxiety or depression. The physical exam should be unremarkable.

The absence of systemic symptoms and no fever rules out IBD.

Bacterial infections are common causes of acute colitis and are usually associated with fever, cramps, diarrhea with tenesmus, and frequently blood in the stool. Common causes of infectious colitis are *Campylobacter jejuni*, *Shigella*, *Salmonella*, and *Yersinia enterocolitica*.

397. **(B)** Review the history to determine if the patient has a lactase deficiency and is unable to tolerate mild products. Patients at risk for lactose intolerance by racial background are Asians, African-Americans, Native Americans, and Jews. It is also important to determine intake of aspartame and sorbitol, which may cause bowel symptoms.

398. **(B)** Antibiotic-associated colitis may occur during antibiotic use or up to 2 weeks after use. Pseudomembranous colitis presents with profuse watery diarrhea with cramps, tenesmus, low-grade fever, and rarely blood in the rectum. Most common antibiotics implicated are clindamycin, ampicillin, and the cephalosporins, though all antibiotics have been implicated. Symptoms usually resolve when the antibiotic is withdrawn, but the disease is potentially lethal and diagnosis should be pursued. Diarrhea occurs secondary to selective overgrowth of the bacterium *Clostridium difficile*, which produces a toxin that causes the lesion of pseudomembranous colitis.

399. **(A)** Order stool for ova and parasites, stool culture, and stool exam for leukocytes to rule out bacterial or parasitic infection. Sigmoidoscopy is recommended when blood or pus is present, or if diarrhea cannot be attributed to a bacterial cause. Barium enema and upper GI series may be indicated. CBC and serum electrolytes would be indicated for evaluation of dehydration.

Ordering the serum alkaline phosphatase and serum amylase would not be recommended routinely in the client's diarrhea workup. The cost of the tests would not be offset by any beneficial effect on the plan of care or assist with the differential diagnosis of diarrhea.

400. **(A)** Classic abdominal pain in appendicitis is moderate to severe and constant and increases with movement. The classic complaint of anorexia often precedes the onset of pain. Other gastrointestinal symptoms are variable (vomiting, diarrhea, constipation). Patient is often afebrile as in this case or may have a low-grade fever. Peak incidence of appendicitis in teens and 20s; it is relatively uncommon in the 40s and 50s.

Acute cholecystitis presents with pain in the right upper quadrant (RUQ) with tenderness and rebound in the RUQ. Pain may radiate to the scapula or shoulder. Most common in women in their 30s–60s. Pain commonly starts a few hours after a large meal. Fatty foods tend to make the episodes of pain worse. Nausea and vomiting are common. Ultrasound is diagnostic.

Ectopic pregnancy is unlikely as the patient's symptoms are not suggestive. The classic presentation of ectopic pregnancy is pelvic pain, adnexal mass, and amenorrhea. Abnormal bleeding, symptoms of pregnancy, and syncope and faintness may also be seen. If suspected, draw an HCG titer and order a transvaginal ultrasound.

401. **(B)** Women present with angina as their initial symptom. Many patients can recall the first incidence of ischemic cardiac pain, although the discomfort is variously described as squeezing, crushing, burning, or heaviness. The pain begins and ends gradually and is usually substernal in location and may radiate to shoulder, jaw, hand, or fingers. Pain may sometimes occur only in a referred location, eg, jaw. The pain of myocardial infarction is diffuse in character and not easily localized.

402. **(A)** The significant subjective feature of ischemia is its predictable relationship to physical exertion, emotional stress, and any activity that increases myocardial demand or decreases oxygenation to the heart. Pain at rest may be diagnostic of unstable angina. Anxiety is a common provocative factor, and the clinician needs to understand the common cycle of anxiety producing chest pain and the pain itself producing heightened anxiety and prolonged chest pain. Angina occurs more commonly in cold or windy weather because of increased peripheral vascular resistance and increased myocardial work. Diurnal patterns may be evident, with angina occurring only in early morning. Heavy meals may exacerbate ischemia. Nocturnal angina may be due to left ventricular failure or may represent unstable disease. Increases in carboxyhemoglobin through exposure to high levels of carbon monoxide in traffic or through tobacco smoke may also increase symptoms.

403. **(A)** The exercise stress test is diagnostic and can be used to assess efficacy of antianginal therapy and extent of myocardium at risk. The goal is to increase oxygen demand and coronary blood flow in a controlled setting. Any obstruction or narrowing of arterial vessels will prevent increased blood flow and result in ischemia. Indications for stress testing include the following: determine the etiology of chest pain, assess prognosis of patients with known ischemic disease, evaluate effects of medical or surgical treatment, and screen healthy middle-aged or older subjects before undertaking a new fitness program and to document response of a patient with known cardiac arrhythmia to exercise and its effect on therapeutic regimens. Adding radioisotopic imaging using thallium-201 isotope will identify occlusive coronary artery disease as well as detecting evidence of a recent remote myocardial infarction with 90% confidence. Thallium scans can also be used to localize the ischemia-producing blood vessel in patients with known coronary artery disease; this information can be helpful in choosing therapeutic regimens.

404. **(B)** Smoking is the major cause of coronary heart disease in young and middle-aged women. Women who smoke have their first MI 19 years earlier than nonsmoking women. Smoking cessation significantly reduces the risk of disease. Risk reduction to that of a nonsmoking woman is not achieved until 3–5 years following cessation. This is independent of the amount or duration of previous smoking. Since this patient has recently quit smoking, she still has the increased morbidity associated with cigarette smoking.

405. **(B)** The Postmenopausal Estrogen/Progesterone Intervention trial studied 875 healthy postmenopausal women in a randomized double-blind placebo-controlled trial over 3 years to test effects of unopposed estrogen and three combined estrogen–progestin regimens on cardiovascular risk factors. Estrogen

alone raised HDL levels more than any of the three combined therapies, but micronized progesterone had a more favorable effect when compared to medroxyprogesterone. This trial does not offer conclusive evidence of cardioprotective effect of hormones. Clinicians need to perform risk assessments on patients and make individual decisions based on these preliminary findings.

406. **(B)** The Tzanck smear is collected from an intact vesicle. The lesion is unroofed and the base scraped and smeared onto a glass slide. The slide is stained with Tzanck or Giemsa stain and sits for 30 seconds. Tap water is used to rinse the stain. The slide is air dried. A microscopic evaluation identifies giant cells and multiple syncytial nuclei. Commercial swabs and viral transport tubes are available for sending the specimen to the laboratory for the staining process.

407. **(B)** The herpes virus resides in the dorsal root or the cranial nerve ganglia following initial exposure to herpes zoster, commonly in the form of varicella (chickenpox). Latent virus may be reactivated at any time and produces a dermatomal or zosterform pattern of vesicles. New lesions may appear for up to 7 days. Lesion duration may be 2–3 weeks. Dermatome patterns that occur most commonly are thoracic, 50%; cervical, 20%; trigeminal, 15%; lumbosacral, 10%. Patients with herpes zoster often develop a prodrome of pain in the affected dermatome.

408. **(A)** When the trigeminal dermatome is affected, involvement may cause lesions of the eye and the patient should be promptly evaluated by a dermatologist. Complications include secondary glaucoma, keratitis, uveitis, and iridocyclitis. Patients are treated with intravenous acyclovir.

409. **(A)** Heberden's nodes are the bony enlargements of the distal interphalangeal joints seen more commonly in women in the fifth and sixth decades of life. The bony prominences are often asymptomatic but a source of concern for the patient. The patient should be reassured

that bony enlargement may not be associated with a degenerative disease process.

410. **(C)** Most patients with osteoarthritis present with pain on passive motion of the involved joint or on motion against resistance. The patient may note crackling or crepitus when the joint is moved. Tenderness along the joint line is common but may be mild or absent. Bony enlargement and irregularity is common, particularly in the hands in the distal interphalangeal joints. There is usually no heat or redness over the joint, although warmth may develop with chronic synovitis.

411. **(C)** Radiographic findings are important in the diagnosis of osteoarthritis. However, x-rays in the early disease stage may be normal. Radiographic findings of joint narrowing and proliferation of subchondral bone with spur formation may also precede symptoms of disease. The more severe radiologic findings seem to correlate with symptoms of osteoarthritis.

412. **(B)** This patient meets several of the major criteria for diagnosing sinusitis, including purulent rhinorrhea for 2 weeks, symptoms of sinus pain, nasal congestion, and a preceding viral upper respiratory infection. Facial pain on bending forward is also found in acute sinusitis. Patients also complain of a cough secondary to postnasal drip; pain may radiate to other parts of the head, neck, or teeth with intermittent fever. Palpation of frontal and maxillary sinus tenderness with the positive findings of the nasal exam support the diagnosis.

Patients with TMJ usually have an underlying dental problem, which may be exacerbated by chewing or jaw movement. History is inconsistent with a classic migrainous headache.

413. **(C)** Patients with sinusitis and no complications can be followed on an outpatient basis. Only patients who do not respond to a treatment course of an appropriate antibiotic should have sinus films to confirm the diagnosis and then be started on a second course of antibiotic treatment. Choice of second treatment would include amoxicillin-clauvulanate (500 mg/125 mg) tid × 14 days or trimethoprim-sulfamethoxazole double strength (TMP-SMX DS) bid × 14 days or a second- or third-generation cephalosporin. Referral is warranted in cases of patients who fail conventional therapy, patients with severe headache and facial pain, and immunocompromised patients.

414. **(A)** Amoxicillin is considered first-line treatment in most uncomplicated cases of sinusitis. It is necessary to use a 14-day regimen to treat adequately; in protracted cases treatment can be extended to 30 days. In the penicillin-allergic patient, the drug of choice would be TMP-SMX DS bid × 14 days.

IV

Professional Issues

Professional Issues Questions

415. Contemporary codes of scientific ethics that safeguard the rights of human subjects are derived from

    (A) The Nuremberg Code
    (B) The Declaration of Helsinki
    (C) A and B

416. The research review committees to protect human subjects are called

    (A) Personnel Review Board
    (B) Institutional Review Board
    (C) Board of Trustees

417. Which of the following statements best describes the purpose of descriptive research designs which use a quantitative approach?

    (A) To examine a single unit under naturalistic conditions
    (B) To generalize research findings
    (C) To study an historical event

418. The advanced practice nurse (APN) obtains her or his legal right to practice from

    (A) The state Nurse Practice Act
    (B) The federal government Nurse Practice Act
    (C) The NP's employer

419. Which of the following best describes the role definition of the Women's Health NP (WHNP)?

    (A) An RN with additional specialized education

    (B) An RN who has practiced for 800 hours in women's health
    (C) An RN who provides care interdependently with the health care team

420. To research the concept of menopause using phenomenology, a qualitative approach, the researcher would

    (A) Survey 3000 randomly selected menopausal women across the country
    (B) Include a culturally diverse population in the sample, which would be representative of all menopausal women's experiences
    (C) Conduct in-depth, open-ended interviews with a small sample to gain an in-depth understanding of lived experience of menopause

421. What is a p value in statistics?

    (A) The probability assuming that the null hypothesis is true of getting a value for the test statistic at least as extreme as the one that actually occurred
    (B) The difference between two sample means
    (C) The probability

422. Which of the following best describes the research variable?

    (A) A characteristic of the subjects you intend to measure or record
    (B) A characteristic of the subjects that varies across studies
    (C) An independent phenomenon

Answers and Rationales for Professional Issues

415. **(C)** Two historical documents set the stage for providing ethical standards of research. The Nuremberg Code or the *Nuremberg Articles,* enacted after World War II, requires informed consent in all cases. The code disallowed any individuals who were not able to give consent. The Declaration of Helsinki (1964 and revised 1974) was published by the World Medical Association for physicians involved in research. As it applies to nursing research, subjects are required to be informed when a clinical or nonclinical study will have no personal benefit.

The following four rights of research subjects must be protected: The right not to be harmed, the right to full disclosure, the right to self-determination, and the right of privacy, anonymity, and confidentiality.

416. **(B)** The Institutional Review Board (IRB) determines that risks to subjects are minimized and reasonable in relation to anticipated benefits. Selection of subjects needs to be equitable. Informed consent is obtained from each subject and is documented. Where appropriate, the research plan makes adequate provision for monitoring the data collected to ensure the safety of the subjects. Adequate provisions must be made to protect the privacy of subjects and maintain the confidentiality of data. Where some or all of the subjects are likely to be vulnerable to coercion or undue influence, such as persons with acute or severe physical or mental illness, or persons who are economically disadvantaged, appropriate additional safeguards have to be included in the study to protect the rights and welfare of these subjects.

417. **(B)** The main purpose of quantitative research is to generalize the research findings. Quantitative research designs involve deductive reasoning, measurement of a controlled or manipulated variable(s), and use of a large sample size.

A case study approach can use a qualitative or quantitative approach. The purpose is to examine a single unit under naturalistic conditions to gain an in-depth analysis of background, environmental characteristics, and conditions. Historiography uses a qualitative approach to study an historical event.

418. **(A)** All nurses and NPs derive their legal right to practice, in the form of occupational licensure, from the states' Nurse Practice Acts. To be licensed as a nurse means that a person has obtained a minimum level of competence in the profession, which requires specialized knowledge (based on academic disciplines). State statutes also recognize to varying degrees that the nurse can act independently and that nursing is a profession that is separate from medicine. Though licensing requirements vary from state to state, most states have regulation specifically for NPs. NPs are typically regulated by boards of nursing, but in a few states joint boards of medicine and nursing or boards related to education of public health regulate NP practice. In the majority of states NPs can write prescriptions and in some states pharmacy boards also may have some jurisdiction. A number of states require that NPs have a bachelor's or master's degree to practice and prescribe.

419. **(A)** The women's health NP is a registered nurse who has successfully completed a formal obstetric-gynecologic/women's health nurse practitioner educational program. This practitioner had acquired special knowledge and skills in health promotion and maintenance, disease prevention, physical and psychosocial assessment, and management of health and illness in the primary care of women. Primary care is provided at all levels of the health care system, but in predominantly an ambulatory setting. The obstetric gynecologic/women's health care NP provides such care in collaboration with physicians as well as other members of the health care team.

420. **(C)** The purpose of qualitative research is to discover, not generalize. Phenomenology is a method that seeks to study the human experience as it is lived. The purpose is to explore a concept (menopause in this case) in depth from women's personal experience. A small n (sample) design is used as the purpose is to gain further understanding of menopause. The researcher is viewed as a participant in the research analysis. Content analysis of transcribed interviews is used to analyze the data.

421. **(A)** The probability assuming that the null hypothesis is true of getting a value for the test statistic at least as extreme as the one that actually occurred is the p value.

422. **(A)** A characteristic of the subjects you intend to measure is the research variable. It results from operationally defining a concept.

Bibliography

Altchek, A. (1993). Dysfunctional uterine bleeding in the adolescent. *The Female Patient, 18*, 45–53.

ACOG, American College of Obstetrics and Gynecology. (1992, July). *Technical bulletin on group B streptococcal infection in pregnancy* (Report No. 170).

Andrews, W. (1995). Continuous combined estrogen/progestin hormone replacement therapy. *Clinical Therapeutics, 17*, 1–11.

Archer, D. (1995). Management of bleeding in women using subdermal implants. *Contemporary OB/GYN, 40(7)*, 1–6.

Association of Women's Health, Obstetric and Neonatal Nurses and National Association of Nurse Practitioners in Reproductive Health. (1996). *The Women's Health Nurse Practitioner: Guidelines for Practice and Education.* Washington, DC.

Austin, H., Louv, W., & Alexander, J. (1984). A case-control study of spermicides and gonorrhea. *JAMA, 251(21)*, 2822–2824.

Barker, L. Burton, J., & Zieve, P. D. (Eds). (1995). *Principles of ambulatory medicine.* Baltimore: Williams & Wilkins.

Barta, A., et al. (1993). Interstitial cystitis. *American Urologic Update Series, 8, XII.*

Bartleson, N. R. (1992). Bacterial vaginosis: A subtle yet serious infection. *Nurse Practitioner Forum, 3(3)*, 130–134.

Baylor College of Medicine. (1995, September). *The Contraception Report. Weighing the Risks and Benefits of Hormone Replacement Therapy* (Vol. VI, No. 4).

Baylor College of Medicine (1995, November). *The Contraceptive Report. Patient Counseling with DMPA* (Vol. VI, No. 5).

Beck, C. T. (1995). Screening methods for postpartum depression. *Journal of Obstetric, Gynecologic, and Neonatal Nursing, 24*, 308–318.

Bird, K. (1991). The use of spermicide containing nonoxynol-9 in the prevention of HIV infection. *AIDS, 5(7)*, 791–796.

Bourinbaiar, A. S., & Fruhstorfer, E. C. (1996). The efficacy of nonoxynol-9 from an in vitro point of view. *AIDS, 10(5)*, 558.

Bourne, T., Campbell, S., Reynolds, K., et al. (1993). Screening for early familial ovarian cancer with transvaginal ultrasonography and colour blood flow imaging. *British Medical Journal, 306*, 1025–1029.

Boyce, J., et al. (1993). Deciding on the interval between Pap smears. *Contemporary OB/GYN NP, 1*, 13–21.

Briggs, G., Freeman, R., & Yaffe, S. (1994). *Drugs in pregnancy and lactation.* Baltimore: Williams & Wilkins.

Briggs, G. (1997). A guideline for treating hyperemesis gravidarium. *Contemporary Obstetrics and Gynecology, 42*, 70–79.

Brody, T. M., Larner, J., Minneman, K. P., & Neu, H. C. (1994). *Human pharmacology.* St. Louis: Mosby.

Caldwell, Jamie. (1996). Hyperthyroidism during pregnancy. *Journal of Obstetric, Gynecologic and Neonatal Nursing, 25 (5)*, 395–400.

Cates, W., & Stone, K. (1992). Family planning, sexually transmitted diseases and contraceptive choice: A literature update. *Family Planning Perspectives, 24(2)*, 75–82.

Cates, W., Stewart, F. H., & Trussell, J. (1992). Commentary: The quest for women's prophylactic methods—hope vs science. *American Journal of Public Health, 82(11)*, 1479.

Chalker, R. (1987). *The complete cervical cap guide.* New York: Harper & Row.

Chuong, J., Otey, L., & Rosenfeld, B. (1995). A practical guide to relieving PMS. *Contemporary Nurse Practitioner, 1*, 31–37.

Chuong, J., Otey, L., & Rosenfeld, B. (1994). Revising treatments for premenstrual syndrome. *Contemporary OB/GYN, 39,* 66–76.

Cotton, D., Horowitz, H., & Powerly, W. (1995). Keeping HIV patients healthy. *Contemporary OB/GYN, 41,* 89–114.

Cramer, D. W., Goldman, M. B., Schiff, I., et al. (1987). The relationship of tubal infertility to barrier method and oral contraceptive use. *JAMA, 257*(18), 2446–2450.

Crumm, C. (1995). Pap smear management. NPACE Conference Cape Cod, MA, July 1995.

Cunningham, F. G., Macdonald, P., Grant, N., Leveno, K., Gilstrap, L., Hankins, G., & Clark, S. (1997). *Williams obstetrics,* Norwalk, CT: Appleton & Lange

Czarapata, B. J. (1996). Interstitial cysitis and vulvodynia. *Advance for Nurse Practitioners, 4,* 21–25.

DeCherney, A. H., & Pernoll, M. L. (Eds). (1994). *Obstetrics and gynecologic diagnosis and treatment.* Norwalk, CT: Appleton & Lange.

Dipiro, J., Talbert, R., Yee, G., Matzke, G., Wells, B., & Posey, L. (1997). *Pharmacotherapy: a pathophysiologic approach.* Stamford, CT: Appleton & Lange.

Dunn, S. F., & Gilchrist, V. J. (1993). Sexual assault. *Primary Care, 20,* 359–373.

Ehrhardt, A. A. (1992). Trends in sexual behavior and the HIV pandemic. *American Journal of Public Health, 82*(11), 1459–1461.

Elias, C. J., & Coggins, C. (1996). Female controlled methods to prevent sexual transmission of HIV. *AIDS, 10*(3), S43–S51.

English, L. E. (1996). Preconception care: A health promotion opportunity. *The Nurse Practitioner, 21*(11), 25–41.

Eyler, A. (1995). Current issues in the care of women with HIV. *The Female Patient, 20,* 15–25.

Fitzgerald, M. (1995). Prescription and over the counter drug use during pregnancy. *Journal of the American Academy of Nurse Practitioners, 7,* 87–89.

Freedman, M., & Nolan, T. (1996). Genitourinary atrophy. An inevitable consequence of estogen deficiency. *The Female Patient, 21,* 62–68.

Freeman, S. (1995). Menopause without HRT: Complementary therapies. *Contemporary Nurse Practitioner, 1,* 40–49.

Friedrich, E. (1983). *Vulvar Disease.* Philadelphia: Saunders.

Galsworthy, T., & Wilson, P. (1996). Osteoporosis. It steals more than bone. *American Journal of Nursing, 96,* 26–34.

Ginsburg, K. (1995). Some practical approaches to treating PMS. *Contemporary OB/GYN, 40,* 24–48.

Glass, R. (Ed). (1988). *Office gynecology.* Baltimore: Williams & Wilkins.

Glazer, H., et al. (1995). Treatment of vulvar vestibulitis syndrome with electromyographic biofeedback of pelvic floor musculature. *The Journal of Reproductive Medicine, 40,* 283–290.

Goldstein, D. J., & Marvel, D. E. (1993). Psychotrophic medications during pregnancy: Risk to the fetus. *Journal of the American Medical Association (JAMA), 270,* 2177–2191.

Grimes, D. A. (1997). *The Contraception Report: Future Barrier Methods and Microbicides,* Emron, 15 Independence Boulevard, Warren, NJ 07659, 3(1).

Harger, J. H., (1997). Genital herpes simplex infections. *Contemporary Obstetrics and Gynecology, 42,* 21–41.

Hatcher, R., et al. (1994). *Contraceptive technology* (16th rev. ed.). New York: Irvington Publishers.

Hawkins, J., Roberto-Nichols, D., & Stanley-Haney, J. (1995). *Protocols for nurse practitioners in gynecologic settings.* New York: Tiresias Press.

Heitman, B., & Irizarry, A. (1995). Hypothyroidism: Common complaints, perplexing diagnosis. *Nurse Practitioner, 20,* 14–19.

Herbst, A., et al. (1993). Interpreting the new Bethesda Classification System. *Contemporary OB/GYN, 38,* 86–107.

Hooten, T. M., Hillier, S., Johnson, C., Roberts, P. L., & Stamm, W. E. (1991). *Escherichia coli* bacteriuria and contraceptive method. *JAMA, 265*(1), 64–69.

Huck, S. W., Cormier, W. H., & Bounds, W. G. (1974). *Reading statistics and research.* New York: Harper & Row.

Iams, J. (1994). Delaying labor with tocolysis. *Contemporary Obstetrics and Gynecology, 11,* 69–71.

International Working Group on Vaginal Microbicides. (1996). Recommendations for the development of vaginal microbicides. *AIDS, 10*(8), 1–6.

Jones, K., & Lehr, S. (1994). Vulvodynia: Diagnostic techniques and treatment modalities. *Nurse Practitioner, 19,* 34–45.

Kaunitz, A. (1993). DMPA: A new contraceptive option. *Contemporary OB/GYN, 38,* 19–34.

Kelaghan, J., Rubin, G., Ory, H., et al. (1982). Barrier-method contraceptives and pelvic inflammatory disease. *JAMA, 248*(2), 184–187.

Kessenich, C. (1996). Osteoporosis cycle. *Advance for Nurse Practitioners, 4*(8), 17–21.

Klaisle, C., & Darney, P. (1995). A guide to removing contraceptive implants. *Contemporary Nurse Practitioner, 1*, 32–43.

Koss, L. (1994). Reducing the error rate in Papanicolaou smears. *The Female Patient, 19* (6), 34–44.

Kreiss, J., Ngigi, E., Holmes, K., et al. (1992). Efficacy of nonoxynol-9 contraceptive sponge use in preventing heterosexual acquisition of HIV in Nairobi prostitutes. *JAMA, 268*(4), 477–482.

Kronberg, M. E. (1995). Down in the dumps. *Advance for Nurse Practitioners, 3*, 31–35.

Kurman, R. J., et al. (1994). Interim guidelines for management of abnormal cervical cytology. *Journal of the American Medical Association (JAMA), 23*, 1866–1869.

Liberman, U., et al. (1995). Effect of oral aldendronate on bone mineral density and the incidence of fractures in postmenopausal osteoporosis. *The New England Journal of Medicine, 333*, 1437–1443.

Lonky, N. M., et al. (1992). Comparison of chemiluminescent light verses incandescent light in the visualization of acetowhite epithelium. *The American Journal of Gynecologic Health, 6*, 11–15.

Louv, W., Austin, A., Alexander, W. J., et al. (1988). A clinical trial of nonoxynol-9 for preventing gonococcal and chlamydial infections. *The Journal of Infectious Diseases, 158*(3), 518–523.

Lynch, M., & Ferri, R. (1997). Health care needs of lesbian women and gay men. *Clinician Reviews, 7* (1), 85–112.

Malolatesi, Catherine R., & Peddicord, Karen. (1996). MTX for non-surgical treatment of ectopic pregnancy. *Journal of Obstetric, Gynecologic and Neonatal Nursing, 25* (3), 205–217.

Manning, F. (1995). Dynamic ultrasound based fetal assessment: The fetal biophysical profile score. *Clinical Obstetrics and Gynecology, 38* (1), 26–44.

Marchant, D. (1994). Risk factors. *Obstetrics and Gynecology, 21*, 561–586.

McKay, M. (1992). Vulvodynia. Diagnostic patterns. *Dermatologic Clinics, 10*, 423–433.

McKay, M. (1993). Dysesthetic ("essential") vulvodynia. Treatment with amitriptyline. *Journal of Reproductive Medicine, 38*, 9–13.

Mead, P., Hiller, S., McDonald, H., McGregor, J., & Sweet, R. (1997). Screening for lower genital tract pathogens in the ob patient. *Contemporary Obstetrics and Gynecology, 42*, 126–145.

Mestman, H. (1997). Hypothyroidism in pregnancy. *Contemporary Obstetrics and Gynecology, 42* (3), 15–24.

Montgomery-Rice, V., & Leach, R. (1993). New options for the diagnosis and treatment of ectopic pregnancy. *The Female Patient, 18*, 31–46.

Munhall, P. L. (1994). *Women's experience.* New York: National League for Nursing Press.

Niruthisard, R. E., Roddy, R. E., & Chutivongse, S. (1992). Use of nonoxynol-9 and reduction in rate of gonococcal and chlamydial cervical infections. *The Lancet, 339* (8806), 1371–1374.

Nolan, T. (1994). Thyroid diseases in the female patient. *The Female Patient, 19*, 81–91.

Nowicki, M., Wax, J., & Balistreri, W. (1997). The maternal–fetal hepatic connection. *The Female Patient, 21*, 46–75.

Paganini, A. (1996). Hormone replacement therapy. *Advance for Nurse Practitioners, 4* (8), 23–52.

Pastuszak, A., Schick-Boschetto, B., Zuber, C., et al. (1993). Pregnancy outcome following first trimester exposure to fluoxetine. *Journal of the American Medical Association (JAMA), 269*, 2246–2248.

Pearlman, M. D. (1995). Management of group B streptococcus during pregnancy. *The Female Patient, 20*, 25–27.

Perkins, R. (1995). The ob-gyn role in sex counseling. *Contemporary OB/GYN, 40*, 27–40.

Plouffe, L., Khreim, I., Rausch, J., & Stewart, K. (1994). Premenstrual syndrome: Update on diagnosis and treatment. *The Female Patient, 19*, 53–60.

Polan, M. (1995). Value of early screening for osteoporosis. *Contemporary Nurse Practitioner, 1*, 19–26.

Prochaska, J. O., et al. (1994). Stage of change and decisional balance for 12 problem behaviors. *Health Psychology, 46*, 13–39.

Rakel, R. E. (Ed). (1994). *Conn's current therapy.* Philadelphia: Saunders.

Redondo-Lopez, V., Cook, R. L., & Sobel, J. D. (1990). Emerging role of lactobacilli in the control and maintenance of the vaginal bacterial microflora. *Reviews of Infectious Diseases, 12*(5), 856–873.

Reece, E. A., Hobbins, J. C., Mahoney, M., & Petrie, R. H. (1995). *Handbook of medicine of the fetus and mother.* Philadelphia: J. B. Lippincott.

Reid, R. (1993). Rational management of cervical and vulvar neoplasia. *Contemporary OB/GYN, 38*, 92–112.

Richwald, G., Greenland, S., Gerber, M., et al. (1989). Effectiveness of the cavity-rim cervical cap: Results of a large clinical study. *Obstetrics and Gynecology, 74*(2), 143–148.

Rodke, G. (1996). Diagnosis and management of vulvodynia. *National Vulvodynia Association News, 1*(4), 1–12.

Rosenberg, M. J., & Gollub, E. L. (1992). Commentary: Methods women can use that may prevent sexually transmitted disease, including HIV. *American Journal of Public Health, 82*(11), 1473–1478.

Rosenfeld, J. (Ed.) (1997). *Women's health in primary care.* Baltimore: Williams & Wilkins.

Sandler, R. S. (1988). Cigarette smoking and the risk of colorectal cancer in women. *Journal of National Cancer Institute, 80,* 1329–1333.

Schieve, L. A., Handler, A., Hershow, R., Persky, V., & Davis, F. (1994). Urinary tract infection during pregnancy: Its association with maternal morbidity and perinatal outcome. *American Journal of Public Health, 84,* 405–410.

Schiffiman, M. (1993). Latest HPV findings: some clinical implications. *Contemporary OB/GYN, 38,* 47–61.

Seidman, S. N., Mosjer, W. D., & Aral, S. O. (1992). Women with multiple sexual partners: United States, 1988. *American Journal of Public Health, 82*(10), 1388–1482.

Seltzer, V. L., & Pearse, W. H. (1995). *Women's primary health care: Office practice and procedures.* New York: McGraw-Hill.

Solomon, D., et al. (1993). 50 years of Pap screening: milestones and missions. *The Female Patient, 20,* 15–19.

Soper, J. (1997). Staging and prognostic factors in gestational trophoblastic disease. *Contemporary Obstetrics and Gynecology, 42* (3), 36–40.

Sosic, A., Hyungkoo, Y., & Chervenak, F. (1996). Transvaginal ultrasonography of the endometrium. Clinical implications. *The Female Patient, 21,* 29–40.

Spadt, S. (1995). Suffering in silence. Managing vulvar pain patients. *Contemporary Nurse Practitioner, 1* (11), 32–38.

Speroff, L., Glass, R. H., & Kase, N. G. (1996). *Clinical gynecologic endocrinology and infertility* (5th ed). Baltimore: Williams & Wilkins.

Star, W., Shannon, M., Sammons, L., Lommel, L., & Gutierrez, Y. (1990). *Ambulatory obstetrics: Protocols for nurse practitioners and nurse midwives.* San Francisco: University of California.

Stein, Z. A. (1990). HIV prevention: The need for methods women can use. *American Journal of Public Health, 80*(9), 460–462.

Stein, Z. A. (1992). Editorial: The double bind in science policy and the production of women from HIV infection. *American Journal of Public Health, 82*(11), 1471–1472.

Stone, K., Grimes, D., & Magder, L. (1986). Personal protection against sexually transmitted diseases. *American Journal of Obstetrics and Gynecology, 155*(1), 180–188.

Tagg, P. I. (1995). The diaphragm: Barrier contraception has a new social role. *Nurse Practitioner, 20*(12), 36–42.

Trussell, J., Strickler, J., & Vaughan, B. (1993). Contracpetive efficacy of the diaphragm, the sponge and the cervical cap. *Family Planning Perspectives, 25*(3), 100–105.

Trussell, J. Sturgen, K., Strickler, J., & Dominik, R. (1995). Comparative contraceptive efficacy of the female condom and other barrier methods. *Family Planning Perspectives, 26*(2), 66–72.

Trussell, J., & Stewart, F. (1992). The effectiveness of postcoital hormonal contraception. *Family Planning Perspectives, 24*(6), 269–273.

van Nagell, J. R., et al. (1991). Ovarian cancer screening in asymptomatic postmenopausal women by transvaginal ultrasound. *Cancer, 68,* 458–462.

Von Gruenigen V. E., & Karlen J. R. (1995). Carcinoma of the endometrium. *American Family Physician, 51,* 1531–1536.

Wilkinson, E. J. (1993). HPV testing—methods and decisions. *The Colposcopist, XXV,* 1–12.

Williams, H. A., Watkins, C., & Risby, J. A. (1996). Reproductive decision making and determinants of contraceptive use in HIV-infected women. *Clinical Obstetrics and Gynecology, 39*(2), 333–343.

Winkleson, E. J. (1992). Adenocarcinoma of the cervix: Evidence of increasing frequency in young women. *The Colposcopist, XXIV,* 1–5.

Winkleson, W. (1990). Smoking and cervical cancer—current status: A review. *American Journal of Epidemiology, 27,* 7–12.

Wright, T., et al. (1993). Managing abnormal Papanicolaou findings. *The Female Patient, 20,* 37–44.

Youngkin, E. Q., & Davis, M. S. (1998). *Women's health: A primary clinical guide.* Stamford, CT: Appleton & Lange.

Index

Genital condylomata, in pregnancy, treatment, 63, 76
Genital self-exam, counseling and education, 10, 36
Genital warts. *See also* Human papilloma virus
  counseling, 11, 38
  diagnostic test, 10–11, 38
  and pregnancy, 11, 38
Gestation
  multiple
    diagnosis, 61, 73
    risk factors, 61, 74
  twin
    dizygotic, 62, 74
    prenatal screening, 62, 74
    prenatal vitamins, 62, 74
    twin-twin transfusion, 62, 74
Glucose level, in pregnancy, 61, 73
Glucose load test, 67, 79
Glucose tolerance test, 68, 79
GnRH-A. *See* Gonadotropin-releasing hormone agonists
Goiter, toxic nodular, Graves' disease vs., 94, 107–108
Gonadotropin-releasing hormone agonists
  for endometriosis, 16, 45
  for leiomyomas, 46
Gonorrhea
  causative agent, 44
  disseminated, symptoms, 40
Graves' disease
  diagnosis, 94, 107–108
  symptoms, 94, 108
GTT. *See* Glucose tolerance test
Guaiac kit, 93, 107

H

Headache
  cluster, 102
  migraine, 88, 102
  Norplant-induced, 8, 34
  tension, 88, 102
Heart disease. *See* Cardiovascular disease
Heart rate, fetal, and twin gestation, 74
Heart sounds, 87, 101
Heberden's nodes, 99, 113–114
Helicobacter pylori
  and duodenal ulcer disease, 109–110
  identification, 96, 110
  prevalence, 109–110
Hemoglobin electrophoresis test, 66, 78
Hemophilus ducreyi, 44
Hemorrhoids
  diagnosis, 97, 111
  treatment, 97, 111
Hepatitis
  alcoholic, symptoms, 92, 106
  diagnosis, 92, 106
  fulminant, 92, 106
  management, 92, 106
  progressive, incidence, 92, 106
  subtypes, 92, 106
  symptoms, 92, 106
  vaccine, allergic reactions, 91, 105
Hepatitis A
  prevention, 91, 105
  transmission, 92, 106

Hepatitis B vaccine
  in HIV-infected patient, 41
  in pregnancy, 66, 78
Herpes simplex virus
  diagnosis, 14, 42, 67, 79
  incubation period, 14, 42
  in pregnancy, 67, 79
  recurrence, 14, 42
  and spontaneous abortion, 67, 79
  treatment, 14, 42
  type 1, 42
  type 2, 42
  virology culture, 42, 67, 79
Herpes zoster
  dermatome patterns, 99, 113
  pain prodrome, 99, 113
  trigeminal lesions, complications, 99, 113
Hirsutism
  and androgen level, 24, 57
  in polycystic ovarian syndrome, 24, 56
Historiography, 119
HIV/AIDS
  and condoms, 33
  immunizations, 13, 41
  opportunistic infections, 14, 41
  prophylactic drug therapy, 13, 41
  risk of gynecologic disease, 14, 41
  testing, 14, 41–42
Hormone replacement therapy
  cardioprotective effects, 99, 113
  management step prior to, 19, 48
Hot flashes, 18, 47
HPV. *See* Human papilloma virus
HSG. *See* Hysterosalpingogram
HSV. *See* Herpes simplex virus
Human immunodeficiency virus. *See* HIV/AIDS
Human papilloma virus
  management, 10, 36
  screening, 9, 36
  subtypes, 38
  transmission, 11, 38, 78
    genital, 38
    vertical, 38
Hunner's ulcer, in interstitial cystitis, 53
Hyperemesis gravidarum, treatment, 63, 76
Hyperprolactinemia, laboratory test, 52
Hyperstimulation, Clomid-induced, 70, 82
Hypertension
  diagnosis, 96, 110
  essential/primary, 76
    diagnosis, 97, 110
    treatment, 97, 111
  intracranial, 8, 34
  laboratory tests, 96–97, 110
  pregnancy-induced, 64, 74, 76
  secondary, etiology, 110–111
  treatment, 96, 97, 110, 111
  and twin gestation, 74
Hyperthyroidism, symptoms, 94, 108
Hypothalamic-pituitary unit, immature, and dysfunctional uterine bleeding, 29
Hysterectomy, for endometrial cancer, 20, 49–50
Hysterosalpingogram
  contraindications, 70, 82
  salpingitis caused by, 70, 82